YOGA
MADE EASY

YOGA
MADE EASY

A personal yoga program that will
transform your daily life

HOWARD KENT

A ☰ People's Medical Society® BOOK

A QUARTO BOOK

Copyright © 1993 Quarto Publishing plc
First published in the U.S. 1994
by the People's Medical Society
Reprinted 1995

Library of Congress Cataloging-in-Publication Data.
      p.   cm.
    Originally published under title: The complete yoga course.
    Includes index.
    1. Yoga, Hatha – Popular works. I. Title.
RA781.7.K453 1994
613.7'046 – dc20   93-46469
                    CIP

ISBN 1-882606-12-4 (trade paper)
ISBN 1-882606-13-2 (hardcover)

The People's Medical Society is a non-profit consumer
health organization dedicated to the principles of better,
more responsive and less expensive medical care. Organized
in 1983, the People's Medical Society puts previously
unavailable medical information into the hands of
consumers so that they can make informed decisions about
their own health care.

Membership in the People's Medical Society is $20 a year
and includes a subscription to the *People's Medical Society
Newsletter.*

People's Medical Society
462 Walnut Street
Allentown, PA 18102
215-770-1670

With special thanks to the models: Adam Benjamin,
Danuta Cockton, Carol Prior, Eamonn Shanahan, and to
Jacqueline Langdon

Typeset by The Brightside Partnership, London
Manufactured in Singapore by Eray Scan Pte Ltd
Printed in Singapore by Saik Wah Press Pte Ltd

CONTENTS

INTRODUCTION

To the question, why should an ancient Eastern concept attract millions of practitioners at the end of the twentieth century?, there is only one answer: because it works.

Yoga offers an attitude to life, from which a variety of practices have developed. First and foremost, yoga produces a feeling of peace, both in mind and body. In turn, this feeling stimulates both thoughts and actions, reminding us of the Latin tag: "Mens sana in corpore sano" ("A healthy mind in a healthy body").

The word "yoga" means unity or oneness – in other words, a feeling of being part of something. Yoga is one of the original concepts which today would be labeled as holistic. That means the body is related to the breath; both are related to the brain; in turn this links with the mind, which is a part of consciousness. The spelling of holistic, too, is a reminder that the word "whole" is derived from "holy" and therefore you cannot be a "whole" person unless you have a "whole" outlook on life itself.

It is not hard to realize that many of our ills today come from the feeling of isolation – *my* problems; *my* pains – a feeling that we are different and separated from others. In the last 50 years there has been a dramatic growth in the understanding of the universal problem now termed "unrelieved stress." At the core of such stress is the feeling of fighting a lone battle against great, often insuperable, odds. Today, thousands of doctors who know little or nothing about yoga nevertheless recommend patients go to a yoga class to help them overcome a variety of stress-related problems. As more research is carried out, so the value of yoga becomes clearer and clearer.

Linking body and mind

Countless exercising plans are available today. New ones come into fashion and then fade away. Almost all of these depend exclusively upon working the body, quite unrelated to the conscious, thinking human being. It would be wrong to say such plans are useless, but their value is extremely limited, because they ignore the proven fact that the mind has a remarkable effect upon the body. Some people quite literally worry themselves to death; while others show a remarkable physical resilience simply because they remain calm and positive. As Buddha declared, some 2500 years ago, "You are what you think."

The aim of this book is to bring together, as simply as possible, the elements which make up life, so that, without making any undue demands, you can find body, breath, brain and mind working as one. It sounds difficult, but because it is a natural process, it is really quite simple once you understand what is happening.

The importance of being able to let go and relax in a world with increasing stress factors has become more and more obvious. Medical research, such as that undertaken in Britain by Dr. Chandra Patel, showing the value of yoga techniques of relaxation in reversing long-held symptoms of high blood pressure, has added a new dimension to the approach of yoga. In the last few years in the U.S., Dr. Dean Ornish has demonstrated that a yoga-oriented program, involving a change in lifestyle, can actually reverse symptoms of heart disease within 12 months. Through these and other important examples, it has become apparent that there is far more to yoga than performing a number of exercises slowly.

Achieving balance

The secret of yoga practice lies in a simple but important word: balance. It has always been stressed that yoga is not for one who eats too little, or for one who eats too much; nor for one who sleeps too little, or for one who sleeps too much. In every area, yoga represents balanced moderation. The idea seems easy enough, but following it through is not so simple in today's complex society. People tend to go at things either like a bull at a gate, or just to play around with them, expecting a great deal of benefit from very little effort. It is all to easy to say: "I don't want any of that philosophical nonsense; I'll just stick to the exercises." Unfortunately, the resulting benefit will be minimal and short-lived. Similarly, it can be just as deceptive to immerse oneself in the philosophy and create a state of mental indigestion!

This book enables you to take the middle path. By starting at the beginning and covering the ground slowly, it offers a program that works for beginners and for relative newcomers. Many people who have attended classes – or are doing so currently – can benefit from having the main elements of yoga outlined and developed in order. One aspect of taking a middle way is to be humble: in other words do not say, "I've done all that – I want to move on," but appreciate instead that it is important to retrace your steps and remind yourself of the basics. Life's lessons need to be learned thoroughly. You should remember, too, that the concept of the middle way applies to how you study, as well as to what you study. The role of the teacher is central, but this role implies not only how and what to instruct, but also how to encourage the student to develop personally both thought and practice.

Many thousands of people attend yoga classes each week, yet seldom, if ever, practice any aspect of the art on their own. Clearly this is unbalanced. The programs offered in this book consist of a series of carefully thought out suggestions. They do not oppose the teachings of a class leader, for there are many ways of approaching this vast subject. What is offered, instead, is a foundation upon which effective practice can be built.

Beware of fundamentalists in all walks of life, including yoga, because they can not appreciate the middle way.

The Purpose of Yoga
Buddha's statement – quoted earlier – "You are what you think," was made 2500 years ago. Around 300 years later, a great sage named Patanjali defined yoga as "controlling the activities of the mind."

The essence of yoga is to be in the driver's seat of life. One of the great British scientists of this century, Sir Arthur Eddington, declared: "The stuff of the universe is *mind* stuff." In other words, real power lies in the mind – the very area that confuses and worries everyone so greatly.

Hatha Yoga
It is easy to make such statements, but much more difficult to put them into practice and, indeed, to live them. Over the centuries a number of interlinked yoga systems have been developed for this very purpose. The system

The Heart Center

most used in the West is called *Hatha* (pronounced "hatta") *Yoga.* Virtually all general approaches come under this heading, although many people put names to their particular approach. Hatha Yoga involves the use of body positions, called *asanas.* (The word *Hatha* is a composite of *Ha* and *Tha*, which are symbols for sun and moon – the actual Sanskrit words are *Surya* for sun and *Chandra* for moon. These symbols signify positive and negative force in the electromagnetic sense; thus *Hatha Yoga* is the yoga of polarized or balanced force.)

In addition to *asanas* the system includes a series of special breathing activities, known as *pranayama.* The translation of *pranayama* is "interruption of breath." In practical terms it involves a series of conscious controls of breathing which provide modifications of internal activities that in turn stimulate or sedate brain activity as required for specific purposes.

Pranayama should not be confused with the enhancement of natural breathing or with the use of the breath in performing the *asanas.* While some *pranayama* techniques are outlined in this book, study of this subject is generally best carried out only under the guidance of an experienced teacher.

Hatha Yoga has a number of other practices not dealt with in this work. These can be studied later because confusion can easily set in if they are attempted too soon.

Hatha Yoga is an introductory system, leading us to greater things. The most celebrated text on *Hatha Yoga* is called the *"Hathapradipika"* (or "Compendium of Hatha Yoga") written in medieval times by a man called Svatmarama. He declared that he taught this *only* for the sake of *Raja Yoga*. The *Raja Yoga* system is specifically to bring about full control of the mind. A raja is the Indian equivalent of a king; thus *Raja Yoga* is called the King of Yogas.

Learning control

Control is a key aspect of yoga: control of the body, breath, and mind. This may seem too much to try to undertake, but what is the alternative? It is to be out of control. This is hardly an attractive prospect and yet, if you stop to consider, the multitude of problems most people suffer from stem precisely from that absence of control.

The *asanas* of *Hatha Yoga*, for example, contain a deep understanding of the principal areas of control of the body, including an understanding of the critical importance of the spine, which not only plays a major role in keeping the body upright, but also provides the vital channel for the nervous system. Keeping the spine flexible, together with working the muscle groups of the trunk effectively, forms a central aspect of yoga postures. Controlled stretching – upward, forward, backward, sideways – and twisting all play a major role.

The result is not simply a more supple and trouble-free back, but also an enhancement of digestive and abdominal organ function and, above all, a natural enhancement of effective breathing – the very core of life itself.

In turn, breathing affects outlook on life, for both oxygen and the body's electromagnetic force are central to effective brain function. Thoughts, attitudes, and emotions are all directly related to the state of body and breath. Agitated, depressed, unhappy thoughts damage breathing while, equally, poor breathing stimulates agitated, depressed, unhappy thoughts!

For almost everyone, life is a series of ups and downs, although we often feel there are far too many downs. You may look for steady happiness but, if you have any sense, you soon realize this is not the pattern of life. Balance, therefore, indicates a situation in which you can make the best of the ups, without trying to cling on to them, and accept the downs as quietly as you can.

Attitude of mind and control
To illustrate a valuable point, try this simple experiment with a friend.

Stand, holding one arm out to the side, clenching the fist to strengthen the muscles. Get the friend to stand behind you, placing one hand on the opposite shoulder to the outstretched arm and the other on the wrist of the outstretched arm. Now the friend firmly, but not jerkily, presses down on the wrist until the arm gives way.

Now put the arm out again and bring into your mind some problem you are currently concerned with, but are having difficulty coping with. Ask your friend to repeat the experiment. You will find that the arm is much weaker.

Put the arm out and once more bring the same problem back into your mind, but say to yourself this time that you know the problem can be resolved and you will not worry about it. The muscles are now much stronger than even at the first trial.

You can, of course, try out the experiment on your friend in the same way. It could be argued that as you have been told what to expect, the result will be a subjective one, so why not try it out on someone without telling them what you believe will happen. You will find that the result is always the same.

Only one factor causes the change in this experiment: attitude of mind. As you have weak thoughts, the body also becomes weak. The brain has conveyed the weakness from mind to body.

Is yoga a religion?

One further aspect of yoga needs to be considered at this stage. Some people claim that yoga can be considered a religion or that it is simply a part of Hinduism, but what are the facts? Yoga, certainly, is not a religion. It has been described as "The art of living, based on the science of living," which is an excellent description.

Thoughts of man's place in the universe, of the concept of God, and of the possibilities of heaven and hell have occupied humanity for countless years. Equally it became apparent that it was easy to *say* something, but far harder really to *feel* it and *live* it. Yoga arose as a series of controls and disciplines in which human beings could begin to experience the principles laid down in spiritual teachings and, by experiencing them, actually to live in accordance with them.

Although not a religion itself, yoga can enhance sincerely held religious beliefs. A number of excellent books have outlined the value

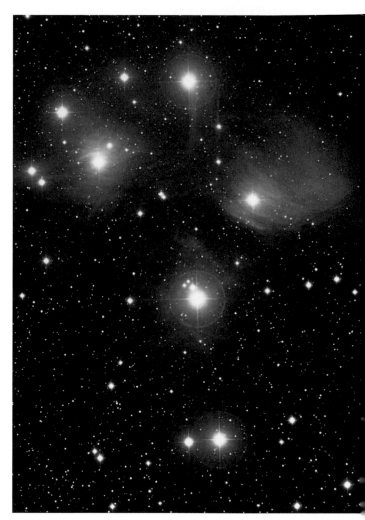

of yoga to Christians, for example. Religious fundamentalists, seeking to claim a monopoly of truth, often denounce yoga, but it is likely that a much greater number of people today would echo the words of Mahatma Gandhi: "Even as a tree has a single trunk, but many branches and leaves, so there is one true and perfect Religion, but it becomes many religions as it passes through the human medium. The one Religion is beyond all speech; imperfect men put it in such language as they can command and their words are interpreted by other men equally imperfect. Hence the necessity of tolerance, which does not mean indifference to one's faith, but a more intelligent and purer love for it. True knowledge of Religion breaks down the barriers between faith and faith."

Yoga, by enhancing true peace of mind, is an effective way of breaking down barriers, mental and physical.

HOW TO USE THE BOOK

There are few requirements for practicing yoga. Clothing should not constrict the movement of the body. Light exercise outfits, such as those adopted for the martial arts, sweat suits, and leotards are all suitable. There should be no constriction at the waist – no belts, for example. It is best to remove wristwatches and jewelry.

Most people like to have their own mat or thick blanket to practice on, but a well-carpeted floor, free from dust, is quite suitable. It is important that your feet do not slip when you do standing poses. A wooden floor is ideal, but not essential. If you find your feet slipping on a carpeted surface, you may want to invest in a thin rubber mat (a camping mat would be fine).

Try to find a spot where you have sufficient room for all the movements. Adequate warmth is important. When relaxing you can cover yourself with a blanket, but avoid anything like a sleeping bag because it will constrict your body.

Naturally, you want peace and quiet. If it is practical, either take the telephone off the hook or switch on the answering machine. Teach yourself not to give in to irritation if you are interrupted; such negative emotions can undo all the benefit you are working toward.

Regular practice
The word "discipline" has unpleasant connotations. Young children traditionally dislike the discipline of washing their necks, yet, if they are obliged to do so, it later not only becomes a habit, but they feel more comfortable and healthier as a result.

The regular practice of various aspects of yoga has the added advantage that the benefits quickly show themselves if the discipline is maintained. There are two most important aspects of the discipline, however. The first is that you must consciously give yourself to the practice, setting aside a period of time and concentrating fully. There is no benefit to be gained from merely going through the motions. In this busy world, people tend to do one thing while thinking or worrying about the next. In this way lie confusion, anxiety, and ill-health. Ten minutes of complete concentrated yoga practice is far better for you than half-an-hour of unsettled thoughts. The second is that you must follow the program best suited to your own needs. It is possible to work to a book or a tape from time to time, but always remember each one of us has different needs. Becoming aware of these needs, and being able to deal with them, is central to yoga.

Yoga and Your Health
The aim of all yoga techniques is to get the best result using the minimum of energy. Because "making an effort" has become so much a part of our contemporary outlook, a number of cautions must be given to those taking up yoga practice.

• If you have any reason to believe you have a condition which affects your health, please seek advice before starting. Consult a qualified yoga teacher or your doctor.

• Those being treated for heart conditions or hypertension (high blood pressure) can benefit greatly from yoga, but should avoid inverted postures and take very seriously the admonitions not to strain to achieve results.

• Forward bending should be avoided by those with a hiatus hernia.

• Asthma and bronchitis can be greatly improved through yoga. Asthmatics should slowly and gently learn to prolong the out-breath.

• Severe lung conditions will cause tissue damage. The stronger breathing techniques should be avoided, but quiet natural breathing should be practiced regularly.

• If you find that any posture causes pain, withdraw slightly. Listen to your body and never strain it.

• Premenstrual tension is countered by yoga, but a woman teacher should be consulted for specific advice.

• There are books available on yoga and pregnancy. There are no general rules because constitutions vary greatly. Again, practical consultation is the best course.

Millions of people all over the world now practice yoga regularly. Over the past 20 years, the Yoga for Health Foundation has not heard of anyone practicing in his or her own home who has in any way damaged his or her own health as a result. On the contrary, countless letters have attested to the benefits which have resulted.

DEVELOPING A PROGRAM

Today, people are invited to follow all sorts of different exercise programs. If any one of these contained "the truth," all the others would fade away; many, however, contain elements of truth that have to be adapted to personal requirements.

The poet Kahlil Gibran encapsulated the proper outlook for yoga when he wrote:
"Say not, 'I have found the truth,' but rather, 'I have found a truth.'
Say not, 'I have found the path of the soul.'
Say rather, 'I have met the soul walking upon my path.'
For the soul walks upon all paths."

In this book, suggestions for building up a regular program of practice are offered at the end of months two to eleven. But these are suggestions only, designed to stimulate study and personal decisions. Some postures, such as the Rabbit, are described but do not appear on the "Continuing the Program" pages. This does not mean that they should not form a part of regular practice, but how they may fit in is a matter for personal decision. To build a program for yourself, take the following factors into consideration:

So far as the physical aspect of postures is concerned, relate to your own body and its needs but do not necessarily regard a disinclination to practice something you find difficult as a message from the body. It is more likely the consequence of a lazy attitude.

Bear in mind the principle of balance, which is at the core of yoga. The need for mental balance can affect which postures you choose to perform. The need for physical balance should determine the order in which they are performed. Many postures are always followed by a counter-posture. For instance, a stretch forward should be followed by a stretch backward.

"Aims for the month" provides a focus for that particular month. Bear that in mind as you learn the new activities for that month.

"Thought panels" complement the activities, providing guidance and stimulating awareness of the interaction between body and mind.

Directory number to indicate month.

Introduction to each month's program. It is important to read this before you start developing your daily program for each month. Remember that these program pages offer a series of examples: the final decision is yours.

Each strand of your yoga practice — postures, breathing, visualization, relaxation, and meditation — has been given a different color.

The pictures act as a memory aid. Refer back to the relevant pages if you need to study the posture or to refresh your memory.

Arrows lead you through the program.

Some postures are paired together, either because you are comparing one with another, or because certain postures are always followed by certain counter-postures.

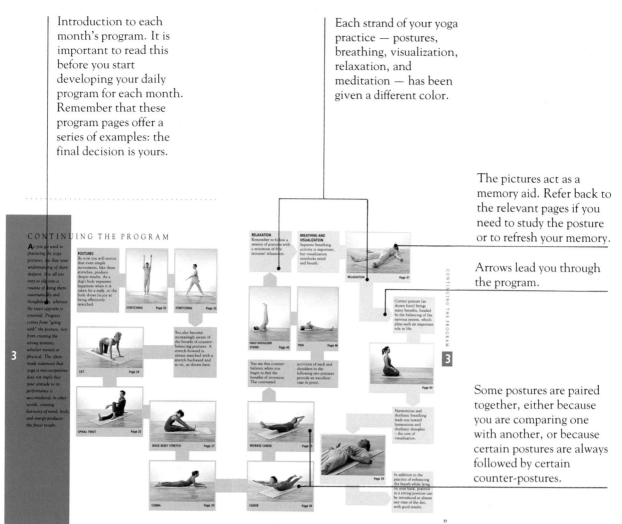

Remember that postures, relaxation, visualization, and meditation are all integral aspects of life. Do not try to mix them up into a salad, but ensure each plays its rightful role.

As you develop a daily program, constantly refer back – right to the beginning. You cannot remind yourself too often of the principles, and the different aspects of practice. Approach the whole business sensibly and happiness, health, peace, and a sense of fulfilment can be yours.

Starting Off

If you can, set aside a specific time each day for practice. Allow at least one and a half hours to digest a small snack or two hours for a meal before you begin. This applies to all postures, including breathing, visualization, and meditation. It is important to allow digestion to proceed unhampered.

The length of your practice will depend on the time you have available and the postures you choose to include in your session. However, it is better to do 10 minutes than to skip practice altogether.

It makes sense to practice each new posture until you can remember the steps without needing to refer constantly to the instructions. It is wise to reread the instructions from time to time to ensure that you are doing the posture correctly and have not left out steps.

Some people may feel comfortable doing the same sequence each day, others will prefer variety. In any case, right from the start, develop the habit of looking through the portion of the book you have studied, remind yourself of the points made, and make your own choice of what you plan to do.

MONTH ONE 1
MAKING A START

MONTH TWO 2
WIDENING THE SCOPE

MONTH THREE 3
MINUTE-BY-MINUTE YOGA

MONTH FOUR 4
MEDITATION

MONTH FIVE 5
BODY AND MIND

MONTH SIX 6
ACTIVE CREATIVITY

1

MAKING A START

AIMS FOR THE MONTH

Slow progression is essential in yoga. Never forget that the central aim is to control the mind and this demands a quiet, methodical approach. Bear this in mind as you tackle the asanas (poses), even though you may feel you can already achieve more than is shown. Content yourself with working within limitations and achieving precise results. If you follow this principle, you will be doing only a small number of things by the end of the month, but you will be doing them well.

• •

FREEING NECK AND SHOULDERS

The first areas of the body to stiffen up are the neck and shoulders. The muscles respond quickly to tension and poor posture, so simple movements to ease these areas should be performed during the day.

• • • • • • • • • • • • • • •

1 Sit looking forward. Breathe in, then breathe out, turning the head to the right. Stop when the breath stops. Breathe in again without moving and again turn to the right on the out-breath.

2 Hold the position and each time you breathe out feel the muscles relax. Breathing in, turn the head to the front and then, on the out-breath, turn to the left, following the same process as in step 1. Let several slow out-breaths relax the muscles.

3 Bring the head to the front again on an in-breath and then, breathing out, drop the chin on the chest. Continue breathing rhythmically and each time you breathe out let the head drop further down, with the chin pressing more into the chest.

4 Breathing in, raise the head and then, breathing out, let it drop backward. Clench the jaw. Continue breathing quietly and every time you breathe out allow the head to drop back a little further, stretching the front of the neck. Finally, breathing out, straighten the head.

5 By combining the breath with a sweeping movement, energy can be pumped quickly into the body. This is an excellent way to get you going when you are feeling stiff or lethargic, especially first thing in the morning. Practice it sitting on the side of the bed or in a chair, or sitting on the floor on your heels. Having breathed out, swing the arms quickly up over the head, breathing in deeply through the nose.

6 Breathing out – also through the nose – collapse forward (but do not over-balance), letting the arms flop down. Release any tension. Repeat eight to 10 times, to stimulate the heart, improve circulation, activate the brain.

STRETCHING

Stretching is important both for health and well-being. It should be carried out quite smoothly and slowly, not jerkily. This routine will tone the nerves and muscles, and improve circulation.

1 Stand erect, feet a few inches apart, palms of hands together, touching the chest. Hold the pose quietly for a minute.

2 Keeping the palms together, bring the hands on the head, with the elbows out. Take a deep, slow out-breath.

3 Breathing in, slowly stretch the arms upward, palms together. Repeat steps 2 and 3 five times, breathing in on the stretch.

4 Next time you stretch up, open the palms forward and raise the arms as high as possible.

5 Then, breathing out, stretch forward, keeping the back as straight as possible.

6 Breathing in, straighten up and swing back, bending the knees to maintain balance.

7 Straightening up, breathe in and stretch to the right on the out-breath, with the arms straight. Repeat the same movement to the left, before once more stretching up as in step 4.

8 Finish by bringing palms together again, back down on to the head, then on to the chest and finally to the sides. Then let the head, shoulders, trunk and arms move freely as you swing from side to side.

THE BREATH OF LIFE

Breath is life, but we also have great voluntary control over our breathing. The key to our energy system is in the diaphragm: a strong sheet of muscle, attached to the bottom ribs, separating the chest from the abdomen. The diaphragm acts as a piston, literally pumping the body's energy.

THE CONTROL OF BREATHING

Breath not only activates the body, it is the basis also of the functioning of brain and mind. Although it is an automatic function, controlling the breath can enhance daily life.

Worry, anger, agitation, and excitement all affect the way you breathe, interfering with the harmony and the flow of energy. Paying sensible attention to the way you breathe is the foundation of effective living.

1

The bottom – or "floating" – ribs are designed to move up and out as we breathe. On the in-breath, muscles open these ribs; on the out-breath, they fall back. Sitting erect on a chair or on the floor, place the hands on the sides of the trunk, covering the bottom ribs. Breathe deeply and slowly and feel the ribs move. The chest and abdomen should be still.

THE SUPPLE SPINE

In the anatomy of human beings, the spine is tremendously important. It provides essential flexibility and support, and it also provides a vital channel for the nerves, while its alignment affects the functioning of important muscles. We allow it to stiffen, or become distorted, at our peril.

When performing yoga movements for the spine, always remember that the body functions as a whole.

1 **The Cat.** Drop on to all fours, knees a little apart, palms facing forward under the shoulder blades. Breathe in, dropping the back and raising the head. Hold for some seconds.

2 Breathing out, arch the back as high as it will go, dropping the head between the arms. Again, hold the position for some seconds. Repeat between 10 and 20 times.

3 Finally, sink back on the heels, hands by the feet, palms facing upward, forehead touching the ground. Remain relaxed for two or three minutes. Get up quietly and slowly.

SPINAL TWIST

Twisting the spine can produce agonizing problems if adequate suppleness has not been maintained. Many people have turned sharply only to spend a long time in a medical corset.

This is a simple, but effective, version of the Spinal Twist. Remember that, by moving slowly and then holding the position, the elasticity of the muscles is enhanced. Sudden, jerky movements are always harmful. Really work the shoulder blades: they will almost always twist round more than you think they can.

1 Sit with your legs out in front of you, feet together, toes pointing upward. Remember to sit upright, lifting the trunk a little, but not stiffly.

2 Bring the right hand to the back, feel where the spine is and bring the palm down on the floor, level with it, a few inches away from the back.

3 Bend the right leg, bringing it over the left leg at the knee joint. Then bring the left arm against the right knee. Breathe in.

4 As you breathe out, swing the shoulders firmly but not quickly, to the right. Close your eyes and hold, breathing rhythmically, for at least 30 seconds. Repeat steps 1–4 on the other side.

THE BACK BODY STRETCH

Back here refers to the whole posterior part of the body. You have to remember that you are constantly subject to the force of gravity. Over the years this can compress the body and needs to be countered by effective stretching.

The Back Body Stretch works from the fingers to the toes: stretching the back of the body and compressing the front of the trunk. The majority of people allow the back to become stiff. The more the mind dwells on stiffness, the greater the problem becomes. Do not regard the pose either as difficult or easy; just say to yourself, "I am doing it," – and follow the instructions carefully.

1 Sit on the floor with the legs out in front, feet a few inches apart, toes pointing upward. Let the hands rest on the floor, palms down by the sides. Breathe slowly out and then, as you inhale, stretch the arms right up in the air, lifting the trunk. This will stretch the spine and the back muscles.

REMOVING STIFFNESS

This is a position which many people find difficult, but if you concentrate on the difficulty you will never progress. In most cases lower-back stiffness comes from lack of use and the muscles are perfectly capable of stretching. The same applies to the hamstrings. Right from the start, perform this *asana* quietly and slowly, and do not let considerations of time affect you.

2 As you breathe out, stretch slowly forward, maintaining the extended back, keeping the arms straight and the back of the legs on the floor. Breath and movement should come together exactly and the only thought should be one of reaching forward.

3 As the out-breath ends, let the hands hold the furthest part they can reach: the toes, the feet, the ankles, or even the calves. Maintain a relaxed stretch with head hanging down. Hold, breathing gently, for at least 30 seconds. Come back up, stretching and breathing in. Then lie and relax.

THE COBRA

Postures in yoga are balanced. Follow the
Back Body Stretch with the Cobra, so that
stretching and compression are complemented.
The Cobra mimics the snake rearing up,
which gives the clue to its performance.
It should seem a natural and inevitable
movement, in no sense should it be straining
for effect. In this way the front of the body is
stretched; both chest and abdomen are opened
up; the back and spine are compressed.
A good way to start is to think of it as a slow,
opening out dance movement, rather like the
petals of a flower unfolding.

1 Begin by lying on the
front, forehead on
the floor, arms by the
sides, palms upward.
Feel comfortable
and relaxed. Breathe
out slowly.

2 As you breathe in,
raise up the head,
neck, shoulders, and
chest. As you feel the
need for extra support,
bring the arms in front,
palms down, to assist
the upward movement.

3 If your back is weak, or there is some muscular or spinal weakness, you can complete the position initially with the forearms resting on the floor. In many cases, however, this will be an interim position. As strength and confidence increase, transfer the pressure to the palms.

1

4 Continue to lift the upper body up, with the arms straight (not bent at the elbow). Adjust the hands to find the most comfortable position. Keep the hips and legs on the floor, so that the arms and trunk balance the upper body. Close the eyes and breathe slowly and quietly. Hold the pose for at least 30 seconds and come down on an out-breath, reversing the movement and then relaxing.

THE ART OF RELAXATION

It is said that relaxation involves the most
difficult asana in yoga. It is called the Corpse
Pose, because it mimics how the body lies
after rigor mortis is over, when all tension
leaves the body. A better name, perhaps is the
Life Pose, because it is wholly open, displaying
neither aggression nor fear. Remember
that relaxation is the opposite of activation.
Therefore, you cannot try to relax. In the
right conditions it will occur spontaneously.

1 Come down
backward on to the
floor with the knees
bent, resting on the
elbows, palms down.

2 Bring the back down
as flat against the
floor as possible, then
slide the legs down, with
the feet well apart.

Relaxation is a process of observation without intervention. First of all observe the breath, which is quite automatic. Say to yourself, "I am not breathing; my body is breathing." Note that the stomach gently rises on the in-breath and falls on the out-breath. Feel the muscles relaxing and that the mind becomes more peaceful as they do so.

You cannot lead a balanced life without periods of relaxation. This is not the same as sleep, which is a combination of restfulness and specific internal activity. Relaxation is the vital process of letting go. While relaxation techniques can effectively be practiced throughout the week, remember the body and mind relax best after some form of physical activity.

3 Move the arms away from the trunk, and roll the palms outward. Let the mind consider the various parts of the body, looking for areas of tension. When practicing relaxation, avoid concerning yourself with time. Initially, the mind is likely to do the opposite, telling you to be up and doing! Don't worry about this; let the process develop slowly but surely. Keep the eyes gently closed and do not lose awareness of the quiet breathing pattern.

WIDENING THE SCOPE

AIMS FOR THE MONTH

During the first month you began to remove tension from the body, learned the vital role of the breath and started to relax. In the second month comes a deepening understanding of respiration and of the power of the mind. You learn to increase the range of movements a little and to start to translate this into a daily program. As you do so, you develop a greater degree of control over how you breathe – and from this you start to see that you can exercise this control over life itself.

• •

ENHANCING THE BREATH

The bottom ribs play a decisive role in breathing (see page 23). Bad posture and agitated thoughts damage the breathing process, but with controlled breathing, the mind and body can be restored.

• • • • • • • • • • • • • • • • • • •

Sit or stand with the trunk upright. Do not slouch or throw the chest out. Become aware of your breath for a minute or two. Then begin to slow it down a little and ensure that it is rhythmical. Place the fingers lightly on the bottom ribs and become aware of their movement. The higher ribs play only a minor role and the abdomen is still. Concentrate quietly on the breath and its rhythmical movement. Be content to continue in this way for two or three minutes.

The diaphragm, attached to the bottom ribs, is dome-like and when you breathe in the movement of the ribs stretches and partly straightens it. This helps the lungs to fill and also creates a vital pressure within the trunk.

As you breathe out, the dome becomes more pronounced again and the pressure is released. This is the essential stimulus both for energy and the natural functioning of the whole of the trunk.

You can enhance this natural breathing process and benefit from it accordingly. Lying down is useful, because it makes the process easier, but the same action can be carried out sitting erect.

Place the heels of the hands to the sides of the rib cage, against the bottom ribs. Concentrate on this area alone and, when you breathe in, let the ribs move out. As you begin to breathe out, firmly without jerking,

press the ribs inward. If they are stiff, be careful but persist steadily. Only if a rib has recently been cracked or damaged is there likely to be any problem. The flexibility of these ribs is an important element of our

energy, mental and physical. Continue the squeeze-and-release process for up to five minutes and then take the hands away and relax for a minute or two before getting up.

ABDOMINAL TONING

In addition to creating a strong, flexible spine, the abdominal muscles must be kept in good condition. Natural abdominal control is essential for effective breathing and it also keeps the glands and organs in good condition.

2

1 The Canoe. Lie on your front, chin against the floor, arms stretched in front, and with the feet close together.

2 Having breathed out, stretch up the right arm and the left leg as you breathe in. Bring them down as you breathe out. Now repeat with the left arm and right leg. Perform each movement three times.

3 Finally, deepen the breathing a little and, as you breathe in, stretch up both arms and both legs, resting on the abdomen. Repeat this three times. Relax for a minute or two when you have finished.

The abdominal muscles can be strengthened by breathing quickly out and, at the same time, pulling the muscles in. Relax them on the in-breath. This can be repeated a number of times. It will help as a preliminary for the Reverse Canoe posture.

UNDERSTANDING RHYTHM

Human life is a series of rhythms. When we are in good mental and physical health, these rhythms harmonize, like the different sections of a symphony orchestra. When they become discordant, when rhythm is lost, we suffer disease (literally, dis-ease), and when we are out of ease, mental and physical difficulties arise. Postures such as those on these pages should be seen from this point of view, not as mere exercises.

The Reverse Canoe.

Lying on your back, feet together, stretch the arms on the floor over your head, bringing the palms together. After breathing out, breathe in and raise the arms, head, shoulders, and legs. Do not bring the hands or feet more than about 15 in. from the floor.

This will maximize the tension on the abdominal muscles. Breathe out as you come down – slowly. Repeat three times, and then relax for a minute or two.

THE PROCESS OF VISUALIZATION

Visualization is a central aspect of human life; we conjure up pictures in our mind's eye all day long. Yoga trains us to take advantage of this natural phenomenon. If applied with concentration, the mind has amazing strength, but, if you simply play about with the idea, results will be only intermittent and unsatisfactory. The ability to retain a simple mental picture can be one of the most important achievements of life. A celebrated Indian yogi, Swami Rama, was involved in experiments at the Menninger Institute in the U.S., where he showed he could control the beat of his heart by visualization.

CONTROLLING THOUGHT

A well-known swami once declared: "Human beings will do anything to help themselves – except to work for it." Once you realize that visualization is a natural, built-in process, you can determine to make it a part of your life. Of course, the brain will keep interposing irrelevant thoughts, but as you persist this will happen less and less. Once you have gained substantial mental control, your life will be enhanced tremendously.

2

Swami Rama simply visualized a blue sky, with small, fluffy almost motionless clouds in it. Because his concentration was complete, the brain accepted this concept as reality and the whole body slowed down accordingly.

To visualize, you do not have to create an actual mental picture, but an impression; the feeling of the picture. Simply as an exercise, sit erect, close your eyes and imagine such a sky: a beautiful summer's day, just a few light clouds and the feeling of peace, warmth, and quiet. If other thoughts intrude, *gently* push them away. This can be repeated whenever you feel like it.

THE RULES OF VISUALIZATION

To visualize effectively, remember that the human framework has developed very specifically. When sitting, we balance on the spine and the muscles need to be harmonized. The spine, too, is important for the working of the nervous system. It is not possible to visualize effectively if you slouch or if the trunk is distorted.

2

1 Unless you can already sit comfortably and correctly on the floor, use a chair. Do not rest against the chair back unless it is upright. Close your eyes, and allow the head to balance comfortably on the shoulders. Wriggle the shoulders a little to ease any tension. Bring the hands together on the lap. Listen to the gentle sound of your breath: feel the cool touch of air on your nostrils as you breathe in and the warm flow of air as you breathe out. Feel the sense of relaxation as you breathe out.

2 Time is now irrelevant. The slow rhythm of your breath is like the comforting tick of a grandfather clock – it enhances the stillness, rather than detracts from it. As you breathe out, repeat to yourself, "I am at peace." When you are truly at ease, gently begin to bring in the visualization you have decided upon. Establish the feeling of it; let it flow all around you. This is to become your reality: you have gone into your own world and are now living fully in it.

A SIMPLE VISUALIZATION

Each breath we take is an intake of energy –
not just from the flow of oxygen through the
lungs, but by the stimulation of the body's
electromagnetic force. In yoga, this is known
as prana. It flows through the nervous
system, stimulates the constant reinforcement
of bone tissue, controls the heartbeat, and
passes messages through the brain. Every cell
in the body has its own electrical field, while
the diaphragm acts as the pump of the
whole system.

Sitting quietly, having checked your posture,
concentrate on your breathing, making it
slow, rhythmic, and peaceful. Visualize your
breath as you draw it in through your nostrils
as a warm, soothing mist spreading as a
warming flow up to the top of the head.
Breathing slowly out, feel the breath flow
through every part of your body, down to the
tips of the toes. If any other thought intrudes,
quietly push it away and let this picture
become totally real to you.

Continue for a minimum of five minutes
(in due course, anything up to 20 minutes).
As you finish, let the visualization fade away,
retaining the feeling of warming energy.
Open your eyes and stretch.

CHOOSING AN IMAGE

In the early stages of
visualization you can get
into the right mood by
recalling a time when
everything felt good.
A vacation perhaps,
where the sense of peace
and the warmth of the
sun united to make you
feel totally in harmony.
Such recollections can
help you create your
own images.

2

DEVISING A PROGRAM

It is important to integrate the various facets of yoga practice into the daily routine of life. Some people say, "I can't afford the time." The reply is: "You can't afford not to."

A major benefit of yoga discipline is that it makes you feel good. That feeling helps the body in all its activities and also makes the mind clearer and more incisive. Half-an-hour spent giving yourself to these practices will save at least a full hour of confusion and stressed activities. ▾

The need for regular practice is not confined to the postures. Helping breathing, calming the mind, promoting peace and health, all have a central role to play.

2

There is much to be said for setting aside a specific time each day for practice, but if this is not possible, then at least try to fit the activities into any time that is available, provided that you allow at least 1½ hours to digest a small snack or two hours for a meal before you begin. This applies to the breathing and mental practices as well as the postures. Allowing digestion to proceed unhampered is important.

POSTURES
Stretching and relaxing form an important preliminary to practicing postures. Stretching should always be counter-balanced by the relaxed swing. Neck and shoulder exercises should also be performed in every session.

STRETCHING   Page 22

STRETCHING   Page 22

The Cat and the simple Spinal Twist provide important toning and enhance the flexibility of the spine. Especially in the early stages, these should be the first spinal movements undertaken.

CAT   Page 24

SPINAL TWIST   Page 25

The Back Body Stretch lifts the trunk to elongate the spine. Avoid a humpy bend as you stretch forward, but equally ease the back into stretching. Then, with the Cobra, make sure that you balance the arms and trunk, so the back can relax without any sense of strain.

REVERSE CANOE   Page 35

CANOE   Page 34

RELAXATION
Relax for at least a minute between all postures which demand the holding of muscle tension. At the end of a posture session, relax for at least five minutes. Most yoga sessions conclude with a relaxation of around 15 minutes.

The Canoe and the Reverse Canoe will tone the abdominal muscles. In the Canoe, legs and arms stretch upward (as shown); in the Reverse Canoe the limits indicated should be followed. In the early stages, watch yourself in a mirror, until you know you are doing it correctly.

BREATHING
Both during a posture session and during the day, pay attention to harmonizing the breath. Ease the rib cage into flexibility, enjoy seeing that your breathing is rhythmical. Be aware of the whole process of energization.

RELAXATION   Page 31

COBRA   Page 29

Page 33

VISUALIZATION
As with breathing, visualization should play a role throughout the day. Do not dwell on the stressful aspects of life – although this does not mean ignoring them altogether – instead promote thoughts of harmony, peace, and beauty. Mind and body will respond.

BACK BODY STRETCH   Page 27

Page 38

MINUTE·BY·MINUTE YOGA

AIMS FOR THE MONTH

The practice of yoga is not merely setting time aside regularly for exercising or relaxation. It is a total approach to living. There is little value in setting brief periods aside for beneficial activities if you slip back into old bad habits the rest of the time. In months 1 and 2, the total interconnection between mind and body has been emphasized. Now that you have practiced some basic movements and glimpsed the exciting mental potential, you can take this integration further.

· ·

RELAXING AT HOME

The word "relax" is often used in two different senses. The yoga sense is letting go by correct use of mind and body; the everyday sense is to flop down. We may not say, "Let's slouch in front of the television," but that is what we do. At meals, also, we all too often hunch our shoulders and crush our digestive system.

· ·

1 Slouching is depleting: back muscles are affected, breathing impaired, and the functioning of digestion and the abdominal organs impeded.

2 Sitting with a thrust-out chest also affects back muscles, can all too easily impede the nervous system, and results in shallow and ineffectual breathing.

Naturally, no one needs to sit correctly *all* the time, but to be effectively active or pleasantly relaxed, correct posture is important. The art of sitting correctly has been a central point of yoga for thousands of years, not just as a discipline, but to allow us to make the most of both body and mind. Many problems can stem – or develop – from "flopped down" evenings.

3 The need for an upright, but not rigid, posture cannot be overemphasized. These pictures are posed in a simple sitting position, but chairs, sensibly used, are just as effective. Sitting well, you are both more mentally alert and are using the body healthily.

MOVING UPSIDE DOWN

The one thing that most people know about yoga is that practitioners often stand on their heads! The Head Stand is not included in this program because it needs careful teaching and, if self-taught, can be harmful. Other inverted positions are easier to learn, and do provide real benefits. The Half-shoulder Stand, for example, improves circulation and blood flow, stimulates the thyroid gland and – when performed in a relaxed manner – takes pressure off the heart.

3

1 The Half-shoulder Stand. Lie on your back, legs together and hands by the sides, palms down. Remember the shoulders will take much of the weight, so make sure they are not tense – wriggle them firmly before beginning. Be aware, too, that you will achieve the position with a comfortable swing from a relaxed body.

2 Having breathed out, breathe in, swinging the legs *and trunk* into the air (legs either bent or straight) as though you were going to roll over on your back.

4 Coming down, use an out-breath, bring the arms, palms down, on the floor behind you to take the weight and *slowly* lower the legs, again, either bent or straight. As the body becomes balanced in each aspect of the *asana*, the whole position becomes both stimulating and peaceful. When you have completed the posture, relax totally for a minute or two.

IMPROVING BODY AWARENESS

The Half- and Full-shoulder Stands are excellent postures for improving awareness of the body. As youngsters we loved to roll on our backs, and we need to recapture this exuberance. A major reason why children have such energy is that they let it flow freely. Adults tend to block or deplete it. The Shoulder Stand, properly performed, is a great energizer.

3 As the legs reach a vertical position, let the hands lightly hold the small of the back. Feel the shoulders rather than the back of the neck taking the pressure. Stretch the toes into the air and then relax the feet. Breathe slowly and rhythmically. Initially, hold for, say, 30 seconds. You will be able to increase this time substantially with practice.

3

THE FISH

*his is the counterpose to the Half-shoulder
Stand, since it compresses the cervical
vertebrae after they have been extended.
It also opens the chest fully.*

1 Lying on the floor
with the feet
together, raise the trunk
on the elbows, arching
the back and letting the
head drop back.

2 Move the elbows
so that the crown
of the head rests on
the floor and the chest
is expanded.

3 Bring the palms of
the hands together
on the chest in the
prayer (*namaste*)
position. Breathe slowly
and deeply. Hold for
about 30 seconds.

VISUALIZATION IN THE POSTURES

The asanas *largely developed from meditative practices. If you hold or use the body in a balanced position and then let your mind dwell on some beneficial concept, the body will naturally adapt itself, becoming more free and supple. This is not easy to achieve, but it brings great benefits. It is one of the unique aspects of yoga, setting it apart from other approaches.*

Regular practice of the postures will ensure that they are performed with the minimum tension and with no waste of energy. As this happens, the visualization aspect can be introduced. Some of the postures you have been practicing should now be coming along well. When you are holding those that feel comfortable and balanced, let your mind dwell on a beautiful sunrise and experience that wonderful sensation of well-being it evokes. You will find that you can hold the posture better and it will be comfortable for longer.

SET YOUR OWN GUIDELINES

Always work with ideas that you find comfortable. For most people a beautiful dawn is inspiring, but a few may have had an unhappy experience that it could awaken. If so, choose another image. Remember, making progress in yoga is a two-way process. Absorb what you are taught, but never forget that you have your own role to play.

3

TAKING STOCK

It is now time to pause and reflect on the progress to date, as well as consider the next steps. Each month has contained some new asanas, but you may well wish that more had been included. The classical language that the sages of yoga used was Sanskrit.
It contains a beautiful word: santosha.
This means being content with where you are and building on that contentment.
It does not mean "putting up with" but rather "working from."

3

Most people embark upon the path of yoga because they want to enhance their life. Everyone needs thoughts to inspire them. For many centuries the sages of yoga have likened human life to the growth of the Lotus flower or Water Lily. The flower is one of the most perfect there is: a circle of beautiful petals glowing on the top of the water of the lake. The Buddhists have a beautiful saying: *"Om mane padme hum"* – "Behold the jewel in the flower of the Lotus." The root of the Lotus, however, is deep in slimy mud at the bottom of the lake. The Lotus root uses these murky ingredients as its nutrients and sends out shoots, which rise in the water until they breast the surface. There – and only there – the bud forms and the perfect flower emerges.

Our lives and the Lotus
Especially in these days of turmoil, our own lives, like the Lotus roots, seem to be submerged and it is easy for us to think that we cannot rise above the problems which surround us. The difficulties and problems that weigh us down are challenges to be faced and overcome; like the Lotus, we can send up shoots that will eventually bloom in the sunshine.

The Heart Center is called the *Anahata Chakra* in Sanskrit. It combines the sun (positive) and the moon (negative) symbols, with 12 Lotus Flower petals around it.

These days we are all too often told we can master important things with very little effort. This is just not true. We can ease the learning process a little but we need *santosha*, and this depends upon developing the power of concentration. Concentration is often talked about and advocated, but few people have the slightest idea of how to achieve it. The specific suggestions offered will help but "If at first we don't succeed…"

3

CONTINUING THE PROGRAM

As you get used to practicing the yoga postures, see that your understanding of them deepens. It is all too easy to slip into a routine of doing them automatically and thoughtlessly, whereas the exact opposite is essential. Progress comes from "going with" the posture, not from creating the wrong tensions, whether mental or physical. The often-made statement that yoga is not competitive does not imply that your attitude to its performance is unconsidered; in other words, creating harmony of mind, body, and energy produces the finest results.

3

POSTURES
By now you will notice that even simple movements, like these stretches, produce deeper results. As a dog's body expresses happiness when it is taken for a walk, so the body shows its joy at being effectively stretched.

STRETCHING　　　　Page 22

STRETCHING　　　　Page 22

You also become increasingly aware of the benefit of counter-balancing postures. A stretch forward is always matched with a stretch backward and so on, as shown here.

CAT　　　　Page 24

SPINAL TWIST　　　　Page 25

BACK BODY STRETCH　　　　Page 27

COBRA　　　　Page 29

RELAXATION
Remember to follow a session of postures with a minimum of five minutes' relaxation.

BREATHING AND VISUALIZATION
Separate breathing activity is important, but visualization interlocks mind and breath.

RELAXATION   Page 31

3

Correct posture (as shown here) brings many benefits, headed by the balancing of the nervous system, which plays such an important role in life.

HALF-SHOULDER STAND   Page 45

FISH   Page 46

You see this counter-balance when you begin to feel the benefits of inversion. The contrasted

activities of neck and shoulders in the following two postures provide an excellent case in point.

Page 43

Harmonious and rhythmic breathing leads you toward harmonious and rhythmic thoughts – the core of visualization.

REVERSE CANOE   Page 35

Page 33

In addition to the practice of enhancing the breath while lying on your back, practice in a sitting position can be introduced at almost any time of the day, with good results.

CANOE   Page 34

MEDITATION

AIMS FOR THE MONTH

The four complementary aspects of human life are activation, relaxation, visualization, and meditation. All are essential to a truly fulfilled existence; all are the basic weapons of health and happiness. You are now using your body in association with the mind and the energy through the breath. You are stimulating your life through relaxation and visualization. Incorporating the peace of meditation is the next major step. In this month you practice more asanas, but, even more importantly, deepen the way in which you use your body, not only when practicing yoga, but also in all aspects of life.

FIRST STEPS

What are the differences between relaxation, visualization, and meditation? In relaxation you allow the body to run, like an idling engine, while you observe but do not interfere. In visualization you use imagery to stimulate the functioning of the body. In meditation you withdraw the mind from the body (without losing awareness of its presence) and dwell on a single, nonphysical concept. This takes you beyond the normal limitations of living, to achieve a much greater sense of control.

You can meditate sitting either in a chair or on the floor. It is not practical to meditate lying down. The conditions already explained (see pages 28–29) apply here: the trunk must be comfortably upright, the hands together (or in a more classical position, in which thumb and forefinger of each hand are touching) and the eyes closed. Some schools advocate meditation with the eyes half-open, but most people find this extremely difficult. It is essential that the body should be comfortable, otherwise messages of distress are signalled to the brain and the calm mental basis is impossible.

There are countless ways of meditating and it is sensible to try several to find one that really suits you, but do not flutter about like a butterfly; that will not be helpful.

Hamsa meditation

An image that has been used for centuries in Indian meditation is that of the wild goose or swan. These creatures are equally at home on land, water, or in the air. As such, they have come to symbolize the free spirit. An effective way to begin meditating is to sit correctly in a room where you will not be disturbed. Close your eyes and bring your mind to the flow and sound of your breath. After a minute or two visualize a goose or swan flying through the air. The Sanskrit word for the bird is *Hamsa*. Keep the visualization for a few minutes and then, as you breathe in, repeat to yourself, "Ham," as you breathe out, repeat "sa." "Ham . . . sa."

Now let the vision of the bird fade, but continue to repeat "Ham . . . sa" together with the in- and out-breath. Any stray thoughts which intrude should be gently pushed away and the chanting resumed. Initially, around 10 minutes is long enough. Gradually you can extend this and, before long, between 20 and 30 minutes will become ideal.

As you get more used to the practice, you will not only find that your mind is both peaceful and alert, but your body will also feel lithe and supple, for the physical benefits of meditation are considerable.

THE MOUNTAIN BREATH

*Initially, we have concentrated on enhancing
the natural process of breathing, because all
too often the pressures and style of daily living
have damaged the way we breathe. Now you
can practice a few techniques that will benefit
both body and breath, and stimulate the flow
of energy. The first of these, the Mountain
Breath, reminds us that the atmosphere in
mountainous regions and areas with rushing
streams is more highly charged with negative
ions, that have been found to be beneficial
both mentally and physically.*

1 Stand, or sit,
comfortably erect,
with the arms by the
sides. Be aware you are
standing tall. Breathe
out slowly.

2 As you breathe in,
stretch the arms,
raising them to the sides,
a little behind the line of
the shoulders, so that, as
they come up, the
muscles of the trunk are
stretched and lifted.

3 When you have
stretched up fully,
link the thumbs and
hold the air in the lungs.
After some seconds,
begin to breathe out,
bringing the arms down,
maintaining the stretch.
Repeat the exercise at
least five times.

4

1 Cleansing Breath.
In these sedentary times, people's breathing is often shallow, and stale air collects in the bottom of the lungs. Offset this by standing erect, feet a little apart, then swing the arms up, bending back a little, mouth closed.

2 Now swing right forward, breathing out through the mouth with a strong "Ha" sound. The head should be loose and the arms dangling. Pull in the abdominal muscles to get more air out of the lungs. Repeat three times.

EXPERIENCING
PRANA

It is all too easy to underestimate the importance of the breath. Literally it *is* life and should be revered as such. When concentrating on the breath – whether to enhance it naturally or by means of specific exercises – the mind should wonder at this Life Force, called in yoga *prana*.

LUNG·CLEARING BREATH

4

LUNG·CLEARING BREATH

Pollution, smoking, and shallow breathing all tend to clog the passages of the lungs, as X-ray pictures show. This exercise squeezes the full lungs to help dislodge mucus and blockages. Anyone with severe chest problems or emphysema should consult their physician before practicing it.

1 Standing as for the Mountain, breathe in, stretching out the arms, bend the elbows and place the fingers on the tops of the shoulder.

2 Retaining the breath, and keeping the fingers on the shoulders bring the elbows to the front.

3 Drop the head and bend forward from the waist, squeezing the chest, still with the breath retained. Hold for several seconds. Then come up breathing out and reverse the initial movement. Repeat three times.

UPSIDE DOWN AGAIN

Is it natural to upend ourselves? You have only to look at children playing to get the answer – they love cartwheels, handstands, and rolling over and over. Keeping the body active and even turning it upside down is a naturally inherited instinct. The inverted positions of yoga rationalize this instinct, to our mental and physical benefit. The Pose of Tranquility is a topsy-turvy posture that is physically stimulating and mentally calming.

While yoga asanas are performed with control, the swing and sense of balance we all had as uninhibited children are essential for effective performance.

4

1 Pose of Tranquility. Lie on the floor, feet together, arms by the sides, palms down. Breathe quite deeply and, on an in-breath, swing the legs into the air, using arms and hands to provide both pressure and balance.

Getting back childish zest
is an important aspect of
adult practice: you need
to combine that instinct
with thoughtfulness.
While the slow,
controlled performance is
central to yoga, you can
often make progress by
first of all coming back to
the roll-about aspect of
childhood and, from this,
impose the greater
control learned as
an adult.

2 When you feel
balanced on the
shoulders, bring up the
arms and hold ankles or
shins. The arms are
straight, not bent at the
elbows. Retain the
position, preferably with
the eyes closed,
breathing gently.
Gradually develop a
floating feeling. Hold it
for as long as is
comfortable. Bring the
arms back to the floor
first to control the slow
lowering of the legs.

3 The Plow.
From the Pose of
Tranquility, you can
move into The Plow
(so-called because the
body resembles a horse-
drawn plow). Remove
the hands from the legs,
lowering the legs until
the toes touch the floor.
Maintain balance by
letting the fingers lightly
support the back. As
with the Pose of
Tranquility, when
coming down, bring the
arms to the floor first
and use them to control
the slow movement of
the legs. Relax for a
minute or two.

4

CONTROLLING OUR RESPONSES

Life is a series of challenges and how people
meet these will over the years play a major
role in their outlook and health. It has been
shown that happy events can challenge people
as much as unhappy ones; all are aspects of
that much-used word, stress. No one can
avoid stressful events, but it is possible to
control reactions to them. Classically, yoga
texts urge that both happy and unhappy events
be treated with dispassion. Few will achieve
this, but it is not difficult to bring about
beneficial modifications.

1 Bad news affects
breathing, which in
turn tenses the
muscles of the trunk.
The flow of energy to
the brain, too, is
impaired, making clear
thinking difficult. If
something bad happens,
sit quietly, place the
hands on the chest,
deliberately slow your
breathing and be aware
of your control both of
breathing in and
breathing out. In a
minute or two you will
feel the pressure ease.

2 Even good news can
upset your
equilibrium. To accept
good news calmly and
effectively, bring the
hands, palms downward
at chest level and feel
you are pushing down
the gasping sensation
which arises. Let the
hands rise a little as you
breathe in and descend
slowly on the out-breath.
Again, ensure that the
breath is slowed.

CHANGING

Reactions to life events become firm reflexes and are hard to change. But change *is* possible and where these reactions are damaging – which is all too often the case – it is important to work to bring it about. For example, the rushing person, always looking at his or her watch and dashing from one thing to the next, can be helped by simply sticking a little colored circle on the watch-face. Every time the watch is looked at there is a reminder of the need to slow down.

3 If something causes worry, you tend to feel that your head is spinning and that you can't quite grasp what is going on. As with all these emotions, conscious slowing and quieting of the breath is essential and, in this case, placing the fingertips gently on the forehead helps to reduce the mental turmoil.

4 Irritating or annoying news can, if not checked, lead to harmful reactions. Bringing the hands on to the chest in the prayer position (*namaste*) has a calming effect, just by its body language. Encourage the breathing to slow and the annoyance will abate.

4

CONTINUING THE PROGRAM

A scientific law, which is also at the heart of yoga thinking, runs as follows: nothing is created, nothing is destroyed, everything is in the process of changing. Any yoga program, too, needs to develop, mature, and change. The emphasis this month moves specifically to the breath. It by no means ignores the postures, but it explores the remarkable enhancement to life that effective control of respiration can bring.

While visualization now plays an important daily role in life, you can begin to explore the wonders of meditation. "Wonders" is, indeed, the word, for meditation can lift you to hitherto undreamed of realms – providing you take it slowly, do not expect miracles, and allow it to develop at its own pace.

BREATHING
However well you advance in yoga, there will always be a place for controlling the breath with the use of the hands.

Page 33

The Mountain Posture combines strong use of the body with valuable development of breathing and this can be linked with the "Ha" breath.

Keeping the lungs clear is of value to everyone, not just those afflicted by chest complaints.

CLEANSING BREATH   Page 55

MOUNTAIN BREATH   Page 54

LUNG CLEARING
BREATH   Page 55

Using these guidelines, you should now be able to devise a breathing sequence of, say, 10 minutes, which will help you in every way.

POSTURES
Practicing a sequence of balanced postures, such as that shown here, will make body, energy, and mind respond. Such a session, even if it is no more than 15 or 20 minutes will leave you glowing.

STRETCHING   Page 22

STRETCHING   Page 22

4

CANOE   Page 34

REVERSE CANOE   Page 35

HALF-SHOULDER STAND   Page 45

COBRA   Page 29

In some ways the Plow is the most demanding pose so far. Its successful performance comes not from striving but from allowing it to happen.

FISH   Page 46

BACK BODY STRETCH   Page 27

PLOW   Page 57

RELAXATION
The final relaxation is becoming more and more important as your physical *asanas* become more demanding.

SPINAL TWIST   Page 25

MEDITATION
Many people are scared of meditation, yet it is a totally natural process. Neither snatch at it nor be afraid of it.

Initially, just feel the joy of letting both body and brain calm down and function quietly.

CAT   Page 24

Page 52

MONTH
5
FIVE

BODY AND MIND

AIMS FOR THE MONTH

People taking up yoga start with a variety of different physical conditions. However, the majority begin with stiffness and some ideas of major limitations. One thing is clear: the body responds to intelligent use. This month you can work a little more deeply towards psychophysical balance. The way you enter into the performance of the asanas will play a major role in determining how well you succeed. It is a good idea to visualize trees and bushes responding to the wind. The graceful movement of the branches suggests a willingness to go with the force.

THE BRIDGE

All postures based on spinal activity also benefit most other parts of the body. Rhythmic massaging of the abdominal organs, for instance, can arise from a combination of movement and breath. Such massage will play a major role in maintaining good health. Meanwhile, spinal flexibility can make a remarkable difference in freeing your body from potential damage.

1 Lie on your back, the arms by the side, palms down, and draw the heels into the buttocks. Breathe out.

2 As you breathe in, raise the back, buttocks, and thighs, and bring the hands into the small of the back, palms open, with the elbows helping to support you. Retain the breath and come back slowly on the out-breath when ready.

PROGRESS IN THE PLOW

Many yoga postures have variations, which provide a further benefit, but their performance is optional. This variation on the Plow position has the unfortunate name of the Choking Pose, but do not let that put you off. There is no need to choke and the development is beneficial!

· · · · · · · · · · · · · · · · ·

The Choking Pose

1 Move into the Plow as previously shown and hold the position for a minute or two breathing quietly. Do not be in any rush.

5

2 Then on an out-breath, bend the knees and bring them onto the floor by the shoulders. Bring the arms around and clasp the hands over the back of the knees by the crown of the head.

Again, hold the position calmly with a gentle breath. Come back into the normal Plow position when you feel ready and, finally, return to the floor slowly on a controlled out-breath. Relax.

SIDEWAYS BEND

1 Stand, legs apart, palms against thighs.

The four basic movements of the spine are forward, backward, sideways, and twisting. The sideways movement is important, not only for the spine itself but also alternately to open up and compress each side of the chest and abdomen. At the same time, the mind, dwelling on reaching out to the right and then to the left, will be calmly focused, helping to improve physical and mental health.

2 As you breathe in, slowly stretch the right arm up, turning the palm inward, until the arm is touching the ear.

3 With the breath retained, stretch the arm up as high as it can go, lifting the shoulder. Breathing out, slowly bend to the left, arm still stretched, until the arm is parallel with the floor. Keep the shoulders parallel with the hips. Hold the position for at least 30 seconds, then reverse the movements and perform the posture with the left arm.

5

64

SPINAL TWIST (LEGS BENT)

Having performed the Spinal Twist with the leg stretched (see page 25), you can move on to a development in which both legs are bent. Each version of the posture has its own value.

Once you have assured yourself that you have got the physical details of postures right, performance depends almost entirely on your state of mind. Do not fuss about the body but dwell on simple, peaceful conceptions. Make sure these are still, or almost so; do not let your thoughts jump about.

1 From a sitting position on the floor, bend the right leg into the groin and bring the left leg over the right knee. The left palm is placed on the floor in line with the center of the back but a few inches from it. Do not lean on the arm.

2 The right elbow comes across the bent left knee, cuddling it into the chest.

3 Breathe in. Then, as you breathe out, firmly twist the shoulders to the left. Keep balanced on each cheek of the buttocks. Close your eyes and feel you are looking around at a beautiful, still scene. Hold for some two minutes, come slowly back to the original position, and repeat on the other side.

5

SPINAL PROGRESS

It is all too easy to continue to perform a
posture regularly without making any mental
or physical progress. Careful, slow progress is
important. This is especially true of asanas,
which are freeing parts of the body that all too
easily tense up, especially the spine, the
muscles of the trunk, and the hamstrings.

5

Back Body Stretch.
Allowing the lower back
to become rigid is all too
common and leads to
much suffering. Do not
forget to lift the back as
you come forward, but
aim to maintain the
stretch without
maintaining a sense of
tension. Above all, do
not be concerned about
time. If the mind is quiet
and the breathing calm
and controlled, the
muscles and joints will
adjust themselves.

Here we take another look at the Back Body Stretch and the Cobra. If, with the Stretch, you have so far managed to hold the ankle or calf, now is the time to aim at reaching the toes. With the Cobra, the straight arms should move in closer, so the spine achieves a deeper curve. In each case, the progress is achieved by allowing it to happen, rather than by grim determination. To succeed, concentrate more completely and ensure that all external considerations are being eliminated.

. . . .

5

CLEARING THE MIND

Start each day's practice with a conscious clearing of the mind. Begin every day afresh. It is all too easy to go through a routine mechanically. One major aspect of Hatha yoga is to bring practitioners into intelligent touch with their bodies, creating true awareness. This is not apprehension, nor is it a form of narcissism. It is, instead, a feeling of belonging, and without it, you do not feel really alive.

The Cobra. With the arms held straight (not bent at the elbows), the arms and trunk are balanced, so there is no undue pressure and the position can be held comfortably. Make quite sure the hips are on the floor, not coming up into the air. The compression in the lower back counters the stretch of the previous posture and strengthens the whole area.

CANDLE MEDITATION

The first requirement of meditation is the power to concentrate – darana in Sanskrit. The realization of this helps you to understand how important meditation is, for everyone knows the value of concentration. The object is to direct the mind to dwell exclusively on one subject. At school, children are urged to concentrate and from then on people realize how important concentration is in order to achieve their goals. Yet, in everyday life, we are seldom taught how to concentrate. Meditation, therefore, offering techniques of concentration, is a valuable aid to all aspects of life, from carrying out mundane daily activities to finding a deep peace of mind.

5

Meditating on a lit candle is a very old practice. It is gentle and calming. It is also a comparatively easy introduction to the art of concentration. Sit erect on the floor or in a chair, having placed the candle a short distance in front of you where you can see it clearly. Gaze steadily at the candle flame for two or three minutes, noting first of all its outline – how steady it is, how it flickers – and then the colors in the flame. Now cover your eyes with your palms and continue to gaze on the image of the candle, which will remain. Continue to note movement and color. As the mind's image of the flame begins to fade, remove the hands from the eyes, keeping them closed, and maintain awareness of the flame even though you can no longer see it. As and when this awareness fades, gently open your eyes. With practice, the final period of awareness will become longer and longer. It can only be maintained through concentration.

USING SOUND

The combination of sound and vision can provide a deep basis for concentration, as we have already seen through the "Hamsa" meditation (see pages 52–3). It has been an Eastern concept for thousands of years that the sound of "Om" (Au-uu-m) is the most sacred of all sounds. It is still chanted daily and, it is claimed, this was the basis of the chant "Amen," used at the end of prayers, hymns, and psalms in Christian services.

In the seventeenth century, the astronomer Johannes Kepler declared that each planet had a "song" and he wrote down the individual notations. A few years ago, a professor of music and a professor of geology in the U.S. took Kepler's laws and notations and applied them to the motions of the planets. This was fed into a computer connected to a music synthesizer. The result was a "song" of the planets – just as Kepler had argued! If planets in motion must project sound, clearly the sum total of all the objects in motion throughout the universe will also provide a sound. One day we may be able to record this, and no doubt, it will be found to be "Om" – the sound of the universe.

As with other forms of practice, the more often you perform this, the longer the periods of total concentration you can achieve. You will find the vibration of this amazing sound brings a feeling of harmony that stays with you.

Again, sitting correctly, with the eyes closed, first pay attention to the calm and peaceful rhythm of your breath. After a minute or two, repeat the sound Om (Au-uu-m) to yourself each time you breathe out. Get swept up in the sound, filling your mind, your body, the room . . . everything with it. If your concentration slips, pay attention to your breath and, after a minute or two, open your eyes.

CONTINUING THE PROGRAM

As you progress, so you grasp the principles more clearly. Yoga is never a matter of learning by rote: it involves getting more and more absorbed in the process so that your individual requirements become apparent. All the different facets are still involved: breathing, postures, relaxation, visualization, meditation – for all are interlinked. Yoga can never be reduced merely to sequences of exercises or techniques. On the other hand, how you blend the elements together will be a matter of personal choice, based on internal awareness.

Before starting your daily program, sit quietly for a few minutes, clear your mind as fully as possible and, slowly but surely, your needs will become apparent.

POSTURES
You are now concerned with development, but this takes place in various ways. Sometimes the new form of a posture will outdate previous performance; in other cases the change is complementary.

Both forms of the Spinal Twist are valuable. Although the earlier one is easier to perform, it provides a really effective twist. The advanced version provides a little more of a challenge, especially if both cheeks of the buttocks are firmly on the ground.

SPINAL TWIST   Page 25

SPINAL TWIST (LEGS BENT)   Page 65

The Choking Pose is a variation of the Plow. Although the advantages of each have been mentioned, as you progress you will understand for yourself what the posture is achieving – or failing to achieve – by listening to your body. This will enhance life in many ways.

COBRA   Page 67

MEDITATION
Meditation benefits you most from being performed every day at the same time and, if possible, in the same place. This is because the brain is happy with reflex patterns; body and brain come to accept it and achieving mental calmness becomes easier. If this is difficult or impossible, just accept that the process will take a little longer. There are many ways in which you can meditate. It is important to find a middle way between experimentation and a jumble of techniques. Proceed quietly and cautiously.

BACK BODY STRETCH   Page 66

Your progress with the Back Body Stretch and the Cobra is a more complete achievement. By practicing steadily and correctly, with the right mental approach, the body eases itself more and more into a truly effective position.

5

BREATHING
All aspects of breathing have a role in your regular program. However, enhancing the natural process and practicing the specific *asana* and *pranayama* techniques should also be integrated into daily life. Correct practice will enable you to "top up" your energy and ensure it flows smoothly. A *pranayama* such as the Black Bee will provide a mental stimulus and can be used whenever you have a few minutes alone.

CHOKING POSE   Page 63

PLOW   Page 57

INSTANT RELAXATION

It is so easy to let things cause you stress that you tend to think it is inevitable, and that you can do nothing about it. Many major problems start with minor ones that go uncorrected and just grow, almost undetected.

Right at the start, the need for stretching, releasing the neck and shoulders and simply swinging energy into the body were emphasized. All these quite simple things need to become a part of life, used when the body signals tension or lack of energy.

Other equally simple actions are shown here in an office setting, but they could be performed equally well in the home or elsewhere.

1 Many activities cramp the body, slow circulation and limit muscle function. To counteract this, work the shoulders and the back for a minute or so, then take the hands and link the fingers as you place them on the back of the head, elbows out.

2 Take a deep breath in and, as you breathe out, press the head down, bringing the chin against the neck and the elbows closer together. Feel the strong stretch on the back of the neck. Hold the position until you feel the need to breathe in again and then release. Repeat at least three times.

Much of our time at work is spent with back and shoulders hunched. This is uncomfortable in the short term and can become serious in time. Apart from the sitting stretch, also perform the standing one already shown (see page 22), even if it is not practical to carry out the whole sequence.

· · · · · · · · · · · · · · · · · ·

It is not always practical to get up and move about; an effective stretch can be carried out while seated in a chair. Link the fingers, letting hands lie on the lap. Breathe in, stretch the arms into the air, turning the hands so that the palms are uppermost. Get the arms level with the ears and straighten them, still stretching up. Hold until the impulse comes to breathe out and then come slowly down. This also should be repeated at least three times.

The biggest problem with simple but important stretches is remembering to do them! The more stiff, irked, and dejected we get, the less likely we are to do anything about it. That is one of the values of a book like this. Keep it where you will look at it regularly. Leaf through the pages day by day and take note of the reminders. After a while a pattern of reflexes becomes established, and you start to reap benefits.

INSTANT RELAXATION

6

BODY AND MIND

Using the body to quiet the mind and enhance inner peace, together with the capacity to act, is a concept little understood in the West. Using the body is considered to be a physical process only and using the mind is not really understood at all. If these two central aspects of life are brought together, your whole outlook changes. You come to realize there is a new dimension to living. The examples given in this book are only "for instances." The one below will probably be something of a surprise, because it is a variation on a standard form of stretching.

6

1 Standing with the legs just a little apart, breathe out and as you breathe in stretch the arms out to the side and over the head. Lift high.

2 Then start stretching up with the right arm, pulling up the whole of the right side.

3 Alternate with the left arm and, after at least a dozen times with each arm, have a final strong stretch up with both arms. Bring the arms down on an out-breath. While performing the stretch fill yourself with a feeling of rejoicing. Liberate the whole body with a joyous feeling.

The Simple Tree.
Mental and physical balance go together, something which is not fully realized. Prayer in India is often combined with physical movements. Today you still see devotees standing on the banks of the Ganges, balanced on one leg, with the hands in the *namaste* (prayer position) on the chest. Their eyes are closed and they are reciting a prayer.

Place one foot on the opposite knee, letting the knee of the bent leg fall outward. Place the hands together on the chest and close the eyes. Repeat to yourself a thought or saying you find helpful, or say a prayer. The length of time you can hold this will increase with practice. Repeat the process with the other leg.

BODY AND MIND

6

CONTINUING THE PROGRAM

Developing a consistent approach to life is of primary importance. Naturally, we all experience many different moods; these will arise for a variety of reasons. Quite apart from events, our outlook is also influenced by fluctuations in our flow of energy and 101 other internal causes. But behind all these factors lies the steady process we call consciousness, and this enables us to bring about beneficial changes when everyday factors make us dispirited, angry, lethargic, or frustrated.

This is why the daily program should never be reduced to a series of exercises. True physical benefit stems from true mental benefit and this is an integration of the different factors that make up life.

No one can see the processes upon which life is based but, although invisible, these life forces *flow*. If we are "open" mentally and physically, that flow enhances our life. Tensions and strains, both in mind and body, block the flow, with highly damaging results.

VISUALIZATION
Visualizing these invisible forces as a golden mist, breathing slowly and calmly, sitting quietly and naturally, enhances all aspects of life. It is combined with postures and should also be carried out regularly on its own.

Page 72

POSTURES
Even simple stretching movements need to be holistic. You can now add the alternate arm stretch to the original sequence. Feel the movements as an expression of vitality.

ALTERNATE ARM STRETCH   Page 76

STRETCHING   Page 22

The Tree and the Mountain have much in common. Steadiness of balance on one leg, with the hands in the prayer position, directs your attention upward. Similarly, the Mountain stretch is an expression of exultation, linking earth and the heavens.

SIMPLE TREE   Page 77

MOUNTAIN BREATH   Page 54

Moving from the Pose of Tranquility, which is largely in the air, into the Plow, which gives the feeling of being grounded, involves somewhat varying moods.

The following two poses always go together. It is useful to perform the simple head and neck exercises first and ensure the shoulders are always flexible.

HALF-SHOULDER STAND   Page 45

FISH   Page 46

SPINAL TWIST (LEGS BENT)   Page 65

SPINAL TWIST   Page 25

The following two poses also go together. Listen to your body: it will quickly show you any ways in which it is unbalanced as well as the ways in which it is being benefited.

BRIDGE   Page 62

Performing the two versions of the Spinal Twist provides a more complete "workout" and helps you to become aware of the effect of similar yet different bodily movements.

BACK BODY STRETCH   Page 66

CAT   Page 24

The flexibility of the back induced by the Cat is a good preliminary to the Bridge.

COBRA   Page 67

POSE OF TRANQUILITY   Page 56

PLOW   Page 57

MEDITATION
Meditation is the king of practices because it takes you beyond the body. This does not mean ignoring the body, but accepting it, while realizing there is something much deeper.

6

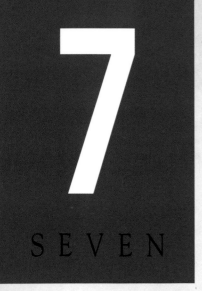

ABOUT ENERGY

AIMS FOR THE MONTH

The human body is a mass of electromagnetic fields, in an electro-magnetic world, which is part of an electromagnetic universe. Some of the body's electric energy is generated by the pumping of the heart, but "no man is an island" and we share this wonderful mixture of waves, vibrations, electromagnetism and gases, which is termed the air or the atmosphere. The term used for it in yoga is prana, which can be translated as "life force." In this month, while keeping up the practice to date, devote your main attention to this force.

THE PSYCHOLOGY OF THE BREATH

Physical and mental stresses and strains will always affect the natural flow of breath, so we will never reach a stage in which we can afford to ignore the day-by-day process.

1 Breath is intimately bound up with every aspect of life. To breathe in, you have to draw the air into the lungs. If you are unhappy, your in-breath is very poor.

2 In the normal out-breath the air is simply allowed to flow out, a relaxed and peaceful movement. A tense person finds breathing out very difficult.

WILLPOWER

↑

TAKING

↑

PHYSICAL STRENGTH

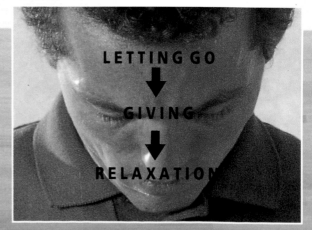

LETTING GO

↓

GIVING

↓

RELAXATION

ENERGY CENTERS

Electromagnetically based energy flows through the body and corresponds with the Chinese concept of acupuncture, now recognized in the West and used by many doctors. The yoga concept is that the body has a series of energy centers, known as *chakras*. (*Chakra* means a wheel or vortex.) These are situated parallel with the spine. While yet insufficiently researched, the evidence for the existence of these centers is growing.

SAHASRARA CHAKRA provides the link between the individual and the universal.

AJNA CHAKRA, the chakra of command links with the hypothalamus and pituitary glands, which order much of our mind-body reactions.

VISHUDDA CHAKRA, in the area of the laryngeal plexus, is concerned with steadiness and balance.

ANAHATA CHAKRA, at the heart center (cardiac plexus) links with emotions over living things ("made my heart flutter").

MANIPURA CHAKRA, at the point of the solar plexus (technically the coeliac plexus) is associated with gastric fire ("fire in the belly") and emotions concerning "inanimate" aspects of life, such as examinations.

SVADISHTHANA CHAKRA is concerned with water, sexual flow, and the sense of taste.

MULADHARA CHAKRA, in the groin area, is related to excretion and the sense of smell.

7

THE ALTERNATE NOSTRIL BREATH

A series of special yoga breathing techniques
go by the Sanscrit name of pranayama.
Literally this means "interruption of breath".
It involves taking control of breathing to
achieve particular purposes. For most of the
time we breathe predominantly through one
nostril or the other. Only for about 20 per-
cent of the time do we breathe equally through
both nostrils. Breathing corresponds with the
positive and negative aspects in electrical
terms. The Alternate Nostril Breath ensures
effective functioning of each nostril and assists
in the balance of energy. It is one of the oldest
pranayama techniques.

1 Bring up the right
hand and close the
right nostril with the
thumb; bend down the
first and second fingers
and place the third finger
by the left nostril.
Breathe in, to a count of
four, keeping the right
nostril closed.

7

2 Close the left nostril with the third finger and retain the breath for a count of 16.

3 Take the thumb away from the right nostril and breathe slowly out to a count of eight. Then reverse the process, breathing in through the right nostril and, after retaining, out through the left. This completes one round. Start with four or five rounds; build up until you can do at least a dozen rounds comfortably.

Another valuable *pranayama* is called the Black Bee. For this, sitting erect, you breathe deeply in and briefly retain the breath. Then very slowly breathe out through the open mouth, making the sound of "ung" – as in "gung". This will sound remarkably similar to the buzzing of the bee, setting up a valuable vibration through the whole body. Repeat at least three times.

THE BELLOWS BREATH

Long ago humans discovered that blowing on a fire caused it to blaze up. For many years they must have been content to use the muscles of their own trunks to achieve this effect. Then, based on their physiological experience, they created the bellows. This directs a strong and beneficial force: the yoga *pranayama* called the Bellows Breath uses that force within the human framework to tone up the system.

Energizing the body
Natural breathing involves tensing the muscles to draw air into the lungs (usually an automatic process) and then releasing them to let the air flow out again. A bellows reverses this process: it expels the air forcefully and then allows it to flow passively in again. Curiously enough, this is akin to the process by which we laugh heartily. A "belly laugh" consists of ejecting the air on the "Ha" sound and then letting it flow back in. The whole process is a fast one, resulting in the body being energized. Not only is oxygen pumped vigorously into the bloodstream, the diaphragm also pumps sharply, stimulating the body's electromagnetic flow. This is why laughter has been discovered to be a first-class therapy, so much so that some hospitals now employ clowns and comics to make the patients laugh.

The Bellows Breath.
This can be performed either sitting or standing. While the back should be erect, it can be tilted forward and the hands placed on the thighs to allow free play to the muscles. Having breathed in, the breath should be ejected sharply through the nostrils, the abdominal muscles contracted to enforce the process. Then the air is allowed to flow back in to the lungs. Having practiced the movements, you can then speed up the process so the breathing becomes very rapid. The sound of the air through the nose on the out-breath will resemble a bellows sound. Somewhere between 10 and 20 such breaths form one round. This should be followed by a slow deep breath in, which is retained for some seconds and then slowly exhaled. Two or three rounds will be quite sufficient, even when one is proficient.

Stimulating the brain
Not only is the body stimulated beneficially in this way, the brain is helped too. We tend not to realize that the brain has a mobile structure; it pulsates. This pulsation directly stimulates mental functions and is affected by the breath. Hearty laughter – or the performance of the yoga Bellows Breath – speeds up the breathing process greatly and this, in turn, stimulates the mental functions. Another breathing process akin to the Bellows Breath is called the Shining Head. The first stimulates the whole body, the latter specifically works on the head and the brain.

7

The Shining Head.
This is performed
similarly, but whereas in
the Bellows Breath the
abdomen is controlled
on the in-breath, in the
Shining Head it is
allowed to expand. As a
result, on the sharp out-
breath the force is more
precisely directed
upward. The many
benefits of these
processes are obvious,
but, as with yoga *asanas*,
the important thing is to
concentrate on the
mental benefits, noticing
the brain clarity that
arises. Circulation, lung
function, and the whole
neuromuscular system
will all benefit.

THE BELLOWS BREATH

7

THE RABBIT

This is a relatively recent yoga practice and is a good way of exercising the three lobe areas of the lungs. It gets its name from the fact that the first two parts resemble a rabbit squatting and sitting up. The third section, sometimes called the Hare, may possibly be thought to resemble a mad March hare. The first movement opens the abdominal area, the second the thoracic (rib cage) area and the third the clavicular (upper trunk) area.

1 Sit back on the heels, with the forearms on the floor in front of the legs, palms downward. Look ahead of you. As you breathe out, quite slowly contract the abdominal muscles, pulling away from the thighs. Breathing in, allow the abdomen to expand, pressing against the thighs. Repeat several times.

2 Now sit up on the heels, hands palms down just ahead of the knees. Again look ahead. Breathing out again, contract the abdominal muscles. This time, on the in-breath the bottom ribs only will expand. Repeat several times.

USING YOUR LUNGS

Using the lungs effectively and keeping them free from congestion is of great importance. Shallow breathing can lead to the lungs holding stagnant air and the passages becoming blocked. Freeing the passageways keeps the lung tissue in a good state and is vital for effective oxygenation of the blood.

3 Bring the hands a little further forward, breathe in and, as you breathe out, bring the crown of the head onto the floor.

4 When the head is firmly on the floor, swing the body forward as you breathe in and swing it back as you breathe out. After several rounds, come slowly up on an in-breath.

RETAINING THE BREATH

Respiration is an automatic process and we are born with reflexes that enable us to adapt the breath to the needs of the moment. But we also have voluntary, or conscious, control of breathing, so that when things go wrong we have the ability to put them right.

By means of quiet intuition and experimentation, yogis realized a long time ago that the control of breathing involves not only inhalation and exhalation, but also the way in which the breath is retained. They called the stopping of the breath *kumbhaka,* and they pointed out that we have the capacity to stop our breathing for a short while after inhaling and after exhaling. They also pointed out that breathing could be brought to a stop at any time and this they regarded as the most important attribute. A central reason for stopping the breath is its effect on the brain and the mind.

When something happens suddenly, causing the necessity of making an instant decision, you stop breathing immediately. If you are driving your car and someone steps out into the road in front of you, you hold your breath without a fraction of a delay. This is because this concentrates the mind totally for a short period while you brake, swerve, or take any other action. Even a delay of a second or so could be fatal.

This instant *kumbhaka* concentrates the mind. Retaining the breath after inhalation helps sedate the mind, putting it into a state of calmness, which enhances the process of meditation.

7

Sit either on the floor or on a chair in a correct position and close the eyes. Breathe slowly and naturally for a minute or two. Take a deep breath in and drop the head so the chin is pressing against the chest. Let the trunk muscles relax so you feel you are sitting on a cushion of air. Keep the breath in and let your mind dwell on a sense of stillness. Do not worry about the breath, just bathe in this state of total nonaction. After a while you will feel the need to breathe again becoming strong. Raise the head, lift the trunk and *gently* breathe out. Let the breathing adjust itself naturally.

Remember that the words for breathing in and out are "inspire" and "expire." Here lies the fundamental balance of existence. The trinity of being is seen in the breath: creation, with the in-breath; preservation, as the breath is retained and, although in one sense breathing out signifies destruction, this is in fact only the process of change. From the breath you rejoice in life and embrace change.

Repeat two or three times, but always take some stabilizing breaths in between.

The length of time you can hold the breath will increase with practice. In the early stages you can check against the second hand of a watch, but give this up as you become more adept. In time you are likely to be able to manage a retention in excess of two minutes.

Remember, this is not a test of endurance but a process taking you toward greater control of body and mind.

Clearly those with heart conditions, or suffering from hypertension, will not attempt this.

7

CONTINUING THE PROGRAM

Conscious concern about the breath involves three distinct approaches. The first is to make sure that the breath is functioning naturally, on the one hand pumping energy through the body and brain, on the other allowing the organism to relax and let go. The multitude of problems, physical and mental, that are endemic in our civilization, disrupts natural breathing patterns.

A second approach is to use the breath in conjunction with movement. In cases such as the Mountain, these become breathing asanas.

The third approach is controlling the breath to produce specific benefits. This we call pranayama.

7

BREATHING
Breath is energy and the diaphragm is the pump involved: using it ensures full use of the lungs and the flow of the body's electro-magnetic force. Becoming aware of the rhythmic movement of the bottom ribs, while the rest of the trunk remains still, is most important.

Page 33

RELAXATION   Page 31

When you relax, the pumping action is greatly reduced. As a result of the relaxation, the abdomen will rise gently on the in-breath and fall slowly on the exhalation. It is important to stay aware of this.

If you want to keep muscles in tone for strong physical or sporting activities, the strong breathing postures, such as the Mountain, are invaluable, because they enhance the electrical flow along the nervous system and build up muscle tone.

MOUNTAIN BREATH   Page 54

POSTURES

It is easy to counsel perfection, but we are not living in a perfect world. There will be days when it does not seem possible to spend more than, say, 10 minutes on postures. Don't think it is not worth it – just concentrate on the four basic movements of the trunk.

These basic movements – stretching forward, backward, twisting and bending sideways – with an opening stretch and a short final relaxation, will provide a mini-session of considerable value. The following poses are just one possible combination; you can develop your own mini-session.

BACK BODY STRETCH   Page 66

A *pranayama* technique such as the Black Bee is very helpful, because it combines control of the breath with a strong vibratory sound. It becomes fascinating to feel how the body responds to the sound and this helps us to understand – and wish to explore – the relationship between vibration, resonance, and health.

COBRA   Page 67

ALTERNATE NOSTRIL BREATH   Page 84

SIDEWAYS BEND   Page 64

Move into *pranayama* techniques with caution. The Alternate Nostril Breath is really the basis of such techniques, because it balances the internal energy system, providing a central role in what is termed homeostasis. However, it should be built up slowly. Both the number of rounds and the lengths of individual components of the breath – in, hold, out – should be increased over a reasonable period. Do not try to do too much, too soon.

SPINAL TWIST (LEGS BENT)   Page 65

CONTINUING THE PROGRAM

7

BRAIN CONTROL

AIMS FOR THE MONTH

Control of physical actions begins in infancy. At the same time, babies start to distinguish sounds and associate them with verbal and pictorial images. As the physical body increasingly comes under control, so the role of the mind is enhanced. Gradually, self-awareness – the link between self and the surrounding world – becomes central to our lives. Yet people all too easily assume that they cannot control their thoughts, although learning to control the brain and to use the mind constructively is the greatest adventure in life. This month the focus is on linking such control with all aspects of life.

COOLNESS AND CREATIVITY

For thousands of years, yoga teachings have insisted that human beings have one aspect of energy or force on one side of the body and a different one on the other, the two interlinking to provide a balanced life. The force on the left side, called Ida, is related to the coolness of the moon and is the calculating aspect of life. That on the right, Pingala, relates to the warmth of the sun and the process of creativity.

In recent years, neuroscientists have established that the left hemisphere of the brain is associated with verbal activity and numeracy – the cool, calculating aspects – and the right hemisphere controls our creative processes – in other words, exactly what the yogis had been saying for centuries.

The brain is divided into two hemispheres: the left hemisphere controls the calculating aspects of life, the right controls creativity.

The importance of balance

Life is a question of balance. Tension, or willpower, is necessary but it must be balanced with relaxation, or letting go. This "letting go" is based upon the in-and-out flow of the breath, upon which all mental and physical functions are based.

Self-awareness, the basis of consciousness, is an instrument by which life can be both developed and enhanced mentally and physically. If, however, you abrogate control of the brain, you abrogate control of life itself; used negatively, self-awareness can become destructive. The choice between creation or destruction lies in our own hands.

Once you are aware, you can use that awareness either positively or negatively. The brain and the body are actually the servants of consciousness.

Creating balance

Bearing in mind the need for balance in all things – sometimes called the middle way – you can review your life and see how far you make use of the cool, logical aspects on the one hand and how far you indulge in creativity in all its forms on the other.

Our present society could well be regarded as left-brain orientated. Once you bring into your life the immense powers of visualization and meditation, and balance tensions with relaxation, you are in a position to contemplate the functions of the brain and to establish the understanding that balance between them is of immense importance. This will, in turn, affect the way you look at many aspects of your life. Beneficial changes then take place, not because you have puzzled about them and calculated them, but because it is part of a natural process.

OVERCOMING RESENTMENT

Medical research has shown that a prime
cause of ill-health – sometimes even death – is
resentment. In overcoming negative emotions,
you do not deny actual happenings, but move
on from them. Visualization can play a major
role in helping to achieve this.

1 Sit quietly and
imagine that you are
with a group of people,
sitting in a circle.
In front of each of you
is a small mound
of modeling clay.
It is plastic, but has
an unpleasant,
muddy color.

2 Pick up the pile of
clay and begin to
mold it with your
fingers. As you do so,
the unpleasant color
reminds you of the
resentments you feel
about people and events,
for such resentments
always feel dark
and heavy.

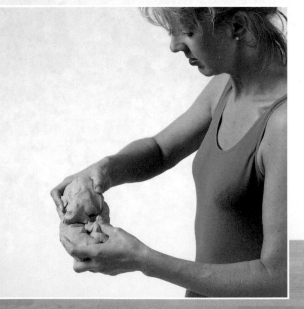

3 Knead your
resentments into the
clay, to bury them in it.
Draw the unpleasant
thoughts from your mind
and squeeze them into
the clay.

4 Finally you – and all the imaginary people around you – make a single pile of the clay on the floor and you realize it contains all your resentments. Imagine that a man with a wheelbarrow comes in, shovels the clay on to the wheelbarrow, and takes it away. You then visualize him digging a hole, tipping all the clay into it, and replacing the soil. You feel a wonderful sense of lightness as you realize your heavy thoughts have been buried forever.

SUCCESSFUL VISUALIZATION

Visualization is like playing a game: to be successful, it demands your whole concentration. Let the scene and the actions be wholly real to you. Although you do not literally have to see the setting, you create an intense awareness of it. The more completely you join in the concept, the more effective the result will be.

8

COUNTERING THE SENSES

The messages our senses provide are thought of as "reality." In fact, sensory reaction is determined by circumstances and habit. For example, in a temperate country, where the temperature was 20°C (68°F), a native inhabitant would regard it as a nice, warm day, a visitor newly arrived from Alaska would find it stiflingly hot, while another from Central Africa would be shivering in the cold. Similar analogies can be provided for the other senses. It is important to realize that the senses are very useful but no one should be a slave to them.

8

Some people become particularly fond of food, for example. At lunchtime their senses remind them a meal is due. The fact that they are well fed and could defer or do without the meal makes no difference. They become unhappy and fret if food is not at hand. Even if there is a good reason for the meal being delayed, they still worry about its absence. The resulting agitation harms the body. In turn, the body feeds back unhappy signals to the brain and a vicious circle begins. In due course, real psychophysical harm ensues. The yoga philosophy develops a spirit of detachment in which the signals of the senses are regarded as useful indicators, but not necessarily as imperative demands. The resulting mental stability, when such a state is achieved, establishes a brain/body harmony that makes for balance, conservation of energy, and enhanced well-being.

State of mind and temperature

In Tibet, where it can sometimes be extremely cold, yogis have shown how they can inure themselves to such conditions, maintaining their body heat. A few years ago, Professor Herbert Benson of Harvard Medical School was able, with the help of the Dalai Lama, to carry out clinical tests on yogis in India. These showed the yogis could select a specific part of the body, such as a finger, and change its temperature by visualization, a process usually described as willpower.

Susceptibility to temperature plays a major role in many people's lives. Although you could adjust the amount of clothing, this is not always possible. Adjusting the state of mind can produce substantial results.

A man living in the Far East found the cold nights very trying and believed he just could not get warm in bed. He consulted a yogi to obtain advice and the yogi told him to visualize a large, glowing ball of golden heat, which came nearer and nearer. He knew that this heat could not singe, burn or hurt him, so he could relax into its rays. He did this every night, and before long his wife moved into another bed, complaining her husband's body was getting too hot!

One effective way of countering a feeling of coolness or cold is to sit correctly, with the eyes closed and recollect a vacation in which you lay on a beach in hot sunshine. If some feeling of cold persists, recall that coming out of the water you have felt a little chilly until the sun has dried your body and again you feel the sun at work. If you do this calmly and with assurance, you will be surprised at the result. You can use the same technique, with a corresponding visualization, to counteract feeling overheated. In both cases, the strength of your concentration will make the brain respond to the visualization, rather than the senses.

8

MIND AND MOVEMENT

The more asanas we perform, the more important it becomes to practice them as an integration of mind-energy-body. Not only does this enhance the performance of the asana itself, it also stimulates the mental processes and will result in an improved quality of life. Every movement can be linked to a mental concept. Once the principles are firmly understood, the visualization can vary, but do not indulge in change for the sake of it. Once you find suitable imagery, it is as well to keep to it, at least most of the time.

The Palm Tree. This is a simple but important posture in which the body is well-stretched above the hips (and legs and hips, too, benefit from the lightening of the load above). It is all too easy to perform this as an unthinking exercise. Resist this temptation.

Stand with the feet 3-4 in. apart, toes pointing to the front. Having breathed out, stretch the arms out to the sides and up until you are reaching as high as you can. Retain the breath as you hold the stretch and breathe slowly out as the arms come down. Repeat several times.

Be the tree while you are doing this. Link the arm movements to a light breeze and the final stretch to the tall tree, reaching up to heaven. Feel the sun and the sense of growth.

Do not be afraid of losing
your balance if you are
drawn into visualization.
Providing you are relaxed,
even if you stumble or fall
you will not hurt yourself.
Damage from falling is
mainly as a result of
tension. In any case this
process will markedly
reduce the chance
of tumbling.

The Tree. You have
already performed a
relatively simple one-
legged posture, noting
that it comes from a
prayer position. Now you
can develop this as an
asana known as the
Tree. Once more the
visualization is that you
are a tree, but this time
you are one with many
branches. In your mind's
eye see the tree on a still
day and then feel you
have become that tree.

Bring one leg up with
the foot into the groin
and let the knee fall
back in line with the
straight leg. On an in-
breath, stretch to the
side and up, finally
bringing the palms
together, maintaining
the stretch. Hold the
breath in until you come
slowly down. Do this,
alternating the legs,
three times each side.

MIND AND MOVEMENT

8

101

A LITTLE FURTHER STILL

The Back Body Stretch and the Cobra were chosen as two basic postures which could be seen to develop over the months. This does not, of course, mean that other postures do not develop in the same way, but by observing the ways in which you stimulate progress with these two, you can apply the same principles to others.

Back Body Stretch. Most people, when they begin to practice this stretch, content themselves with holding their ankles and calves. Before long they find they can hold their toes. Now is the time to explore the capacity to link the hands around the feet.

Remember that everyone's body is built differently and do not force the movements. However, with the right approach, great progress can be made. Make sure that as you stretch the arms up on the in-breath, you elongate the back and open up the spine as fully as possible. Make sure you do not lose this stretch as you begin to breathe out and move forward. The movement should be as effortless as a drawbridge coming down. Tension in the mind can put an undue strain on the lower back muscles and this can be damaging.

The stretch forward and down should continue the feeling of well-being. The more you enjoy this, the better the muscles and joints will respond.

8

Always remember that in a very real sense the body wants to be used. Many medical practitioners confirm that one of humankind's major problems is called "disuse atrophy," or "If you don't use it, you lose it." There may be specific physiological reasons why you cannot perform certain postures fully, but don't fall back on the excuse that you are stiff.

• • • • • • • • • • • •

In today's frenetic society, everyone lets themselves be dominated by time. The result is we achieve less, fail to do things properly and damage both mind and body.

If you lose yourself in postures such as these, the energy flows freely, the body benefits and you are stimulated mentally. You can get much more done in a day if you do each thing fully. These postures can be immensely helpful in this respect.

The Cobra. The same principles apply here. The back will follow the stretch to the front of the trunk and you will find the palms can move closer in, remembering at all times to keep the arms straight, with no bend at the elbows. If the legs and hips take the weight, the balance becomes comfortable and you can appreciate the sinuosity of the movement.

A LITTLE FURTHER STILL

8

103

There are many people only too ready to tell you the "right way" to do something, although there is rarely a specific "right way." Some yoga teachers extol the virtue of performing each sequence every day. Others urge variety.

It is important to realize that what is offered in these pages is a series of examples: the final decision is yours. This decision should arise from tuning in more and more to the requirements of body and mind.

It takes some time to distinguish intuition from inclination. Avoid giving in to the "I don't feel like it today" syndrome, but realize that this feeling may direct you to a program that meets the specific need of the moment.

8

POSTURES
The Tree offers an interesting posture development. The Simple Tree is a prayer – or meditative – position; the second a more specific balanced stretch. Do not, however, lose the meditative value in attempting the more advanced posture. Concentrate on balance, not imbalance; realize how much the mind directs the body.

SIMPLE TREE   Page 77

TREE   Page 101

ALTERNATE ARM STRETCH   Page 76

STRETCHING   Page 22

Spending some time on different aspects of stretching helps to clarify the advantages and to explain why apparently similar movements will produce a variety of results. If you clear your mind and accept the feedback, you will find significant differences.

MOUNTAIN BREATH   Page 54

PALM TREE   Page 100

BREATHING
When clearing the air in the lungs with the "Ha" breath, add a further dimension by remaining down after the third exhalation. When no more air can be expelled, breathe gently through the nose and bend the arms, so that each hand holds the opposite elbow.

Page 37

Chronic pain can be diminished, even eradicated, by processes similar to the one with the clay. Develop the feeling that you do not need the discomfort and that you are taking it out of your body and placing it somewhere else, where it cannot return to you. The key to success lies in the degree of concentration.

VISUALIZATION

Remember that there are countless ways of visualizing. Provided you follow the basic rules, you can introduce your own concepts. Always be erect, always let the breath be quiet and rhythmic, and keep the eyes closed and the hands together on the lap.

Page 97

CLEANSING BREATH Page 55

CLEANSING BREATH Page 55

MEDITATION

Pranayama techniques control the breath to control the mind. Once you have practiced retaining the breath, this can be used as a preliminary to meditation. Breathing in, sitting on one's "cushion" of air and retaining the breath for a minute or so will, once you are used to it, induce a feeling of calmness. Follow immediately with a short period of meditation.

Continue to breathe rhythmically and feel the head and shoulders come down a little as you breathe out. Let this be a natural stretch – do not tug. After two or three minutes, drop the arms again and, on an in-breath, straighten up, swinging the arms over the head and bringing them down by the side on the out-breath. This will enhance the suppleness of the lower back muscles.

Page 90

Page 52

DEVELOPING
ASANAS

AIMS FOR THE MONTH

By now it will be obvious that you are developing quite slowly as far as the asanas are concerned. This is deliberate; it is better to learn to do a few things well, rather than a lot indifferently. Many people take up exercise programs and other systems that offer all sorts of techniques, but very few keep them up for long, primarily because the techniques are superficial. By its clear, slow integrated progress, yoga becomes a way of life and every aspect of living is enhanced as a result. This month you continue to bind all the strands of yoga together.

STANDING BACK AND BODY STRETCH

Touching the toes is an exercise everyone performs as a child; some keep it up much later in life. However, most tend to "snatch" at it, thus jerking the neuromuscular system, often doing more harm than good.

1 Stand with the feet about 12 in. apart, arms by the sides. Breathe out, and, on the in-breath, swing the arms, quite slowly, into the air, lifting the trunk.

2 On the out-breath, swing forward, continuing to stretch and come down as far as you can, with the arms hanging.

If possible, let the fingers touch the floor, preferably, place the palms on the floor. Shake the head a little to make sure you are not holding tension in the neck. Breathing gently and slowly, hold the position for a minute or two, lengthening the time with practice.

Come up on an in-breath, reversing the whole process carefully and finish by bringing the arms to the sides as you breathe out.

3 To counter the forward stretch, link the fingers behind the back and, as you breathe in, swing back with the arms well away from the buttocks and with the knees a little bent.

4 As you breathe out, come slowly back to the original position. Repeat steps 3 and 4 three times.

9

THE TRIANGLE

A *sideways bend was introduced earlier (see page 64). This was a relatively simple but effective movement that can certainly be retained in the program. The best-known classical sideways bend posture is the Triangle, which you now move on to. The shoulders must remain parallel with the hips throughout. There is usually a tendency to twist the shoulders in order to achieve more, but this is wrong. The extent of the stretch can be improved gradually.*

1 Stand with the feet quite wide apart (about 18 in.), the toes of the right foot pointing out at right angles, those of the left pointing slightly to the right. Breathing in, stretch the arms out to the sides.

2 As you breathe out, bring the right hand against your thigh and slide it down the calf while you lift the left hand into the air, turning the palm to face the front.

3 Look up at the hand in the air and let the right hand rest on, or hold, the ankle. Breathe quietly and hold the position. (In due course you may find you can place the right hand on the ground behind the foot.) When ready, come up on an in-breath, reversing the movement. Perform three times on each side.

IMPROVING

For an effective sideways bend, imagine you are an inverted pendulum. Before doing the posture, it can be helpful to swing the trunk. Not only is this bend helpful to the spine, it balances the many functions within the trunk, and also balances the muscle groups. Such spinal movements are particularly useful to people who play sports such as golf, tennis, and racketball, that tend to exercise one side of the body only.

THE TRIANGLE

9

THE BOW

The Bow is a strong posture and those who are not naturally supple may find it difficult. For such people – a considerable majority – it is an interesting challenge in slowly but surely letting things happen rather than striving after them. To perform this posture effectively, a change in the normal approach to breathing is important.

1 Lie face down, with the feet together, head on the floor and the arms by the sides, palms up. Breathe out.

2 Breathing in, hold the feet with the hands and bend the legs so the heels come in to the buttocks.

3 Breathe out, then breathe in again and, exactly at the moment you breathe deeply out, lift the head, shoulders, and chest, and pull on the feet to lift the calves and thighs off the floor, so that you are resting on your abdomen. Hold the out-breath and then come gently down again before breathing in. Repeat three times. Making the movement on the out-breath ensures that the strong pull is made on relaxing muscles.

9

THE BOAT

This is a suitable counterposture to the Bow.
It requires an overall sense of balance.
Although many of the body's muscle groups
are put in tension, minimum effort is needed.

1 Lie on the back, feet
together and arms by
the sides, palms down.

2 Breathe out and, on
the in-breath, swing
the legs, straight into
the air.

3 Stretch the arms in
front of you. Finally,
swing the trunk up, so
that you are resting on
the base of the spine, the
arms outside the legs.
Come down by reversing
the movements on an
out-breath. Repeat
three times.

THE BOAT

9

DEEPENING RELAXATION

Although the relaxation position has been shown and practiced, it has not so far been analyzed in detail. This is because you first have to become accustomed to relaxing in this way and then you can begin to remove pockets of tension. Relaxing is deceptively difficult because it involves letting go, and "trying to relax" is a contradiction in terms. On these pages you can see the main areas where tension is apt to be retained. After consciously working on these for a while, the body adjusts itself automatically and only rarely will it be necessary to go through the trouble spots.

Feet. When lying in relaxation the feet should be well apart, about 12-15 in. This helps the leg muscles to relax. The ankles, too, need to relax, so the feet flop outward.

Back. Many people will find that when they are lying there is a gap between the lower back and the floor. This can be minimized by bending the knees, so the heels come into the buttocks, and by gently sliding the legs down again, at the same time consciously pressing the lower back against the floor.

Hands. The arms should lie well away from the trunk and the hands rest comfortably, palms upward, not downward. It can be helpful to wave the hands and wrists loosely and then let them flop on the floor.

Head. The head should be in a straight line with the body, with the chin neither pressed in nor pulling away. A shake of the head will free the neck muscles and the shoulders should be consciously pressed against the floor and then relaxed.

DEEPENING RELAXATION

9

MORE STRENGTHENERS

Many people fail to realize that yoga asanas strengthen the body in a natural and effective way. This is a very different approach from body-building or similar techniques and it works equally well for both men and women.

It is not part of yoga to create bulging or rippling muscles, but the essential strength of all parts of the body is improved considerably as part of a balanced program.

The Mountain Breath.
This exercise, which you have already been practicing, combines deep use of the lungs and diaphragm with an upward stretch of the muscles of the trunk and arms. This variation involves a more lateral movement.

Sitting or standing, let the arms fall by the sides, palms and fingers open. Breathe deeply out and, on the in-breath, begin to stretch the arms out and up. As the arms come above the shoulder blades, begin to bend them until each hand is firmly gripping the opposite elbow. Make sure the arms are well back, in line with the back of the ears. Hold the position, keeping the breath in. When the impulse to breathe out becomes strong, begin to do so slowly, reversing the movement, until the arms are again by the sides. Repeat five or six times.

1 **The Lion.** This may look ferocious, but its aim is to provide an extremely strong therapeutic pressure, balanced by the subsequent relaxation. Sit erect with the hands on the knees or thighs and take a deep in-breath.

REGULAR RELAXATION

The strength involved in yoga *asanas* is always balanced. What everyone needs is the capacity to act strongly when the necessity arises, not to live in a permanent state of tension.

Regular moments of relaxation play a central role in yoga: everyone needs to remind themselves of this balance to enjoy a harmonious life.

2 Breathe strongly out through the wide open mouth, expelling the air with a loud "Ha" sound. At the same time, protrude the tongue until the tip touches the chin, and glare intensely at the tip of the nose, while tensing the fingers, hands and arms. Gradually let the muscles relax. Repeat three times.

The Tongue Lock. This exercise also provides strong balanced pressure. Sitting erect, breathe in through the nose. Holding the breath, force the mouth open wide, with the tongue placed limpet-like on the upper palate, until it comes away with a clicking sound. Repeat a number of times.

MORE STRENGTHENERS

9

115

THE PEACE OF UNITY

The activities of the human brain are so
remarkable that you can hardly begin to
appreciate them. Many thousands of signals
are processed every second. Even when you
are in the state of dreamless sleep, the brain
continues to record and take in the
appropriate automatic action. But the brain is
the servant, not the master.

Once you take a step toward the mastery of
your own mind, you also take a step toward
a feeling of internal peace. When you begin to
calm the mind through meditation, you find
that the brain is constantly feeding you stray
and irrelevant thoughts and sensations. Often
the best way of handling these is to push them
away, gently and purposefully, so that you
can return to a state of concentration.

Stray thoughts   **Feeling of touch**

Apprehension of taste   **Perception of sounds**

PEACEFUL ACCEPTANCE

While pushing away ideas that are not required is often desirable, it can be just as successful to practice accepting them.

Try sitting quietly in the meditative pose, breathing slowly and gently, letting the feeling of calmness sweep over you. Then, when the brain begins to turn, accept the messages, even welcome them. Pay attention to each stray thought. Note carefully every sound. Become aware of any sensation of taste. Appreciate the feeling of touch: the clothes against the skin, the body against the floor.

The result will be similar to what happens when a naughty child tries to goad his or her parents into reaction. The more the child succeeds, the worse the problem becomes; the more the parents note, but do not react to, the child's naughtiness, the more the child feels a sense of anticlimax. Teasing is no fun anymore and before long he or she gives up.

Letting the brain/mind know that you will accept or ignore its messages as you wish plays a significant part in helping to quiet it, and also in stimulating a deep internal feeling of well-being.

The various approaches to mental control should not be kept simply for specific sessions. Many a problem can be resolved by switching off for a short period – even a minute or two – before tackling it again. In the right surroundings and the right weather, we can all feel peaceful, but when you feel a sense of peace during periods of noise or confusion, you know that you are making progress.

Whenever you sit quietly, in meditation, visualization or even in relaxation, take note of your face. Body language involves the way in which the facial muscles are used: not only do people screw their faces up against bright light, the wind or some other phenomenon, but they tend to do so in relation to problems. Become aware of your brow and allow any furrows to drop out. Relax the muscles around the eyes. Let the mouth and jaw be slack and make sure the tongue, too, is not tensed up against the palate. This simple process will be a positive aid to calmness, and it will also make you look younger and more attractive.

CONTINUING THE PROGRAM

This month we focus on some stronger postures. Remember that such postures in yoga are not "show off" activities. If you find some of them beyond you, despite being in the right mental state and having advanced carefully and slowly, do not worry. Work away gently, but do not allow yourself to feel irritated, frustrated, or upset: these emotions are damaging and will obstruct your goal.

Try to be dispassionate, and simply accept that this is your degree of performance for today. Remember, too, that human bodies vary considerably physically and that what is easy for one person is extremely difficult for another. Accepting genuine limitations is as important as overcoming mental inhibitions.

POSTURES
You have now advanced from a simple Side Bend to the classical Triangle. Both are still valuable. Never discard simple things: they all have their value. Do not fall into the trap of wanting to be "advanced." True humility is important.

SIDEWAYS BEND   Page 64

TRIANGLE   Page 109

STANDING BACK & BODY STRETCH   Page 106

STANDING BACK & BODY STRETCH   Page 106

Having concentrated earlier on the sitting Back Body Stretch, we now introduce the standing version. The combination of a genuine stretch with a relaxed state of mind remains vital. Muscles will bear a remarkable load if they are encouraged rather than tugged at.

It is important to keep practicing the earlier Back Body Stretch and the Cobra. You will notice the improvement in your ability to perform these poses as the months pass.

BACK BODY STRETCH   Page 102

COBRA   Page 103

9

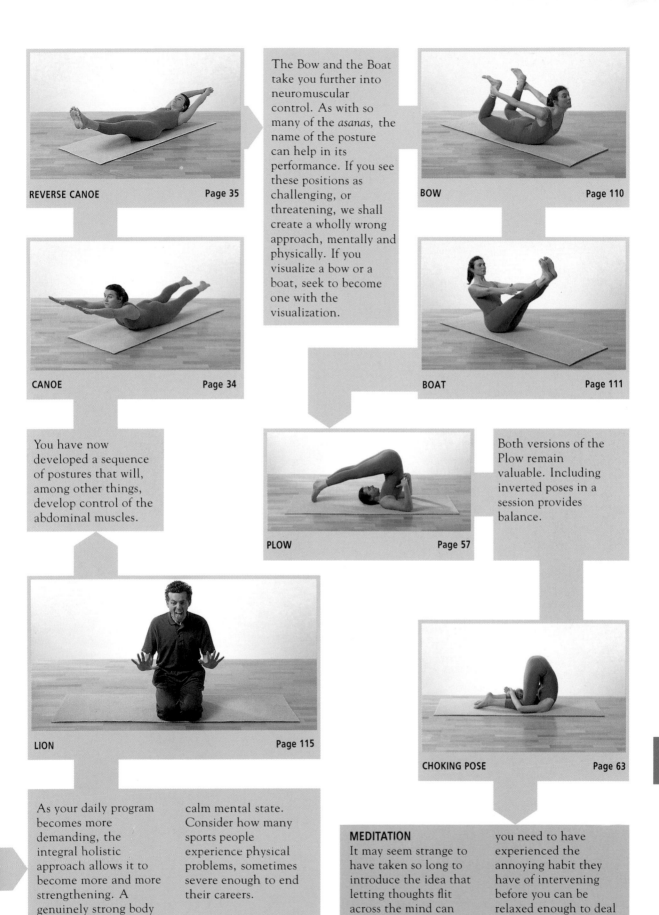

REVERSE CANOE   Page 35

The Bow and the Boat take you further into neuromuscular control. As with so many of the *asanas*, the name of the posture can help in its performance. If you see these positions as challenging, or threatening, we shall create a wholly wrong approach, mentally and physically. If you visualize a bow or a boat, seek to become one with the visualization.

BOW   Page 110

CANOE   Page 34

BOAT   Page 111

You have now developed a sequence of postures that will, among other things, develop control of the abdominal muscles.

PLOW   Page 57

Both versions of the Plow remain valuable. Including inverted poses in a session provides balance.

LION   Page 115

CHOKING POSE   Page 63

As your daily program becomes more demanding, the integral holistic approach allows it to become more and more strengthening. A genuinely strong body arises from a genuinely calm mental state. Consider how many sports people experience physical problems, sometimes severe enough to end their careers.

MEDITATION
It may seem strange to have taken so long to introduce the idea that letting thoughts flit across the mind can help you to clear it, but you need to have experienced the annoying habit they have of intervening before you can be relaxed enough to deal with them in this way.

TEN

PROPORTION

AIMS FOR THE MONTH

The more involved you become with a subject, the more you take it seriously. In many ways this is excellent, but you need to keep a sense of proportion and to ensure that fun and lightness never lose their role. This is, after all, only another example of the need for balance. You are now nearing the end of your opening year, and it is time to leaven the progress with effective lightheartedness. The leading exponents of yoga in India – the swamis – all have a great sense of humor. This month, therefore, progress – both mental and physical – is maintained through knowledge, practice, and enjoyment.

THE HULA HULA ASANA

This makes no pretense of being a yoga posture, but possibly the only reason it isn't is climatic. People living in hot climates tend to be more supple than those in the colder zones; their bodies are not always tensing up against chill winds and pouring rain. Westerners need to counter the weather's effect.

1 Stand with the feet apart and place the hands on the hips.

2 Begin to gyrate the hips, as though doing a sexy dance or keeping a hula hoop in the air.

3 Sense the rhythm, speed up, slow down, and at all times make the wiggle as wild as you can – have fun doing it. You will find your breathing adjusts itself to the movement.

If done with a sense of fun, this exercise will liberate the lower back, not only making it easier to perform the classical *asanas* for the spine, but also improving general suppleness. If it is performed too earnestly, the tension could pull a muscle; so let go and enjoy yourself. It's great to be a child again.

10

THE HANUMAN POSES

Hanuman, *king of the monkeys, plays*
a beneficent role in Indian mythology.
These strong poses combine the use of the
breath with effective control of the muscles.

1 Lunge forward,
making sure there is
a good bend at the knee
joint. Stretch the arms
in front, parallel with
the shoulders, with the
palms downward.
Take a deep out-breath.

2 As you breathe in
strongly, swing the
arms up over the head.
Keep the lunge position
and hold it until you feel
the urge to breathe out.
Repeat three times. Now
change to the other leg.

3 Lunge again, as in 1, but this time, as you breathe out, bring the clenched fists together (thumbs inside) with the knuckles almost touching.

4 Once again breathing in strongly, swing the arms outward so the chest is well expanded. Again hold the position; repeat three times and then change to the other leg. Repeat three times again.

The essential element of sitting correctly is the erect back. One of the images that most people associate with yoga is the Lotus Position, in which each foot rests on the opposite thigh. Children find this simple to do, but adults find it more difficult. When practicing sitting postures, it is important to remember the knee is a hinge joint – it is not designed to rotate. Therefore it must be used carefully. The Lotus is best taught on a one-to-one basis, and many people can advance well in yoga while still only sitting in a relatively simple cross-legged position. With gentle but persistent practice this can become balanced and comfortable.

1 To improve the cross-legged position, sit on the floor and take one ankle in both hands, while the other leg is bent in to the groin. Now use the hands to lift the ankle, while the leg muscles seek to pull down the knee. Practice for a few minutes with each leg. The movement needs to be rhythmic, not jerky.

2 Now bring the soles of the feet together and bring the hands around the feet.

SITTING CORRECTLY

There are many views on the correct way to sit on the floor in yoga. If you intend to do so for some time, it is sensible to place a folded-up blanket or a cushion under the buttocks.

While discomfort is often felt in the early stages, if you proceed correctly you will be rewarded with a growing feeling of comfort. Eventually you wonder how you came to sit any other way.

3 Holding the feet, move the knees up and down. This is often called a "butterfly" movement. You will feel the strain in the groin area, but if you maintain the rhythm and the feeling for the butterfly-like movement, the muscles will slowly accept the pressure and stretch sufficiently. When you have done this for two or three minutes, keep the soles of the feet together but place one hand on each knee and gently but firmly push it downward. It will not be long before you notice a distinct improvement.

SITTING COMFORTABLY

10

BUILDING UP ENERGY

Energy, the be-all and end-all of existence, was discussed on page 83, where we pointed out how much misunderstanding there is about the matter. Oxygen plays a central role in human life, but it is not essential to all life. According to the philosophy of yoga, there has to be some basic force that is universal and upon which countless permutations are built. The ancient yogis called this force prana; the Chinese called it chi; Bergsen called it elan vital. Generally, it is translated as Life Force. You have already been practicing working with this force: now, with the aid of a friend, you can experience it more precisely.

1 The natural breathing process is for the bottom ribs to move up and out on the in-breath, stretching the diaphragm, and to fall back on the out-breath, the abdomen and chest remaining still. Some people claim that, to use the lungs effectively, the abdomen should also expand and contract with the breath.

10

The two forms of breathing shown allow the lungs to be used equally well, so the changes in strength cannot be caused by oxygen. The difference comes from stimulating the electrical flow down the nervous system, a factor discovered many years ago. Breathing naturally, therefore, you generate your own electrical force, upon which all other aspects of energy depend.

Most youngsters have natural poise and breathe as nature intended. Our way of life, with its tensions and pressures, knocks this out of us quite early. Once you have restored the natural posture, you can improve the breathing. To start with you need to practice, even if only briefly, quite frequently. This will be recorded on a "floppy disk" in the brain – in other words, you establish a reflex action that will come into force as required.

2 Get a friend to help you and, before you begin, put one arm out to the side, tense the muscles, and ask your friend to push it down firmly. Take half a dozen deepish breaths, allowing the abdomen to expand as you breathe in. Now get your friend to check the tone of the arm muscle once more. It will have gone quite weak.

Next, take a similar number of deepish breaths with the abdomen and chest still and the bottom ribs moving out and back (as you have been practicing already). Get your friend to try once more: your arm will have strengthened markedly.

BUILDING UP ENERGY

10

127

CONTINUING THE PROGRAM

It is not possible to impose feelings of vitality, peace, joy – they all come from within. The "Continuing the Program" pages are a memory aid rather than detailed working sheets. If attention this month is centered on sitting, it does not, of course, mean that steady practice of all the other aspects should be abandoned.

People who know little else about yoga have often heard of the Lotus position, which involves placing each foot on the opposite thigh. When we were young children, most of us could do this easily, showing that it is in no way unnatural. However, as we grow up, the nature of the lives most of us lead makes us in some ways stiffer and stiffer.

As a result, the Lotus is not offered in this book. Those who can achieve it without damaging the knee joints are free to do so, but it is only one of a number of effective sitting positions.

POSTURE
Sitting, standing, and walking upright are natural activities for humankind, central to body design or development. As a result, an upright posture is the most comfortable way, for everything is in balance.

Page 83

Bad posture distorts the body, putting wrong strains and pressures on joints, ligaments, muscles, and so on. This physical distortion is reflected in the brain, which passes on the messages of discomfort to the mind. This discomfort is not merely registered physically, it also begins to damage our outlook generally.

Page 72

Page 42

Taking time to restore good posture is important in every way. Attention to standing posture is important, but it will tend to follow the posture we adopt when sitting. Getting that right is therefore of primary importance.

10

Sitting on the heels is quite simple. If the muscles in the ankles have tensed up, they will stretch back quite easily if they are trained in short, steady bouts. The feeling of discomfort will disappear quite soon in the majority of cases.

Page 43

Sitting cross-legged on a cushion or folded blanket is generally advisable. The muscles in the groin will also relax considerably if they are allowed to do so. Remember, they can be encouraged to do so with gentle hand pressure.

Page 38

Page 116

SITTING
You can sit effectively in any reasonably well-designed chair. If the back of the chair does not provide good support, sit up and do not lean against it.

Once you have acquired the art of sitting and standing naturally, any other position seems irritating and uncomfortable.

10

MONTH

11

ELEVEN

CENTERING – BECOMING ONE

AIMS FOR THE MONTH

An often used expression when mind and body are not functioning together is "out of sync." In this state it is easy to break things or misjudge distances; you cannot "think straight" and breathing becomes disturbed. There are, of course, prosaic explanations of what is happening, but normally no one knows why. At this point in your practice, a simple understanding of human synchronization is important.

THE BODY'S SHEATHS

The yogi sees the body as made up of a series of sheaths, superimposed one on the other. When life is balanced and harmonious, these fit together closely and life functions as a coordinated whole. However, all too often the layers do not fit together and life becomes "disconnected." There are five of these sheaths; the first is the physical body, nourished by the food we eat; the second is the air we breathe, without which there is no life; the third, the storage and coordination functions of the brain; the fourth, the mental process, which gives us the opportunity to discriminate and exercise free will, even if this is only to a limited degree; the fifth is the link with universal consciousness, which results in many people having an occasional glimpse of oneness, an ecstatic moment.

It is helpful to build up the realization of the various layers of consciousness that make up a human being. All aspects of yoga are directed towards the creation of an harmonious whole.

The sheaths can form an ideal subject for contemplation when you are sitting quietly, but there is no reason why you should not bring them to mind at other times. Just being aware of them is a step towards balance.

Thinking about the complexity of existence is helpful. While you can hardly begin to understand it, the realization that you are immersed in a sea of waves, vibrations, and resonances will help you in the vital process of knowing that you are a part of an immense whole, rather than an isolated unit.

11

THE TRIPOD

This inverted posture looks difficult, but it isn't, provided that instructions are followed carefully and the various aspects of your being are allowed to function together. It is, in fact an ideal posture to ensure that the five human sheaths are functioning together.

1 Come down on all fours, with the arms straight, palms down and facing forward at shoulder level and at shoulder width.

2 Place the crown of the head on the floor so that it forms the apex of an equilateral triangle, with the hands as the bottom corners. Be quite sure you have the triangle right.

3 Bend the arms so that they are at right angles at all points. Place the right knee on the corresponding elbow.

4 Place the left knee on the corresponding elbow and balance comfortably breathing calmly and allowing the mind to maintain the quiet decision to hold the posture. Retain it for as long as you are comfortable.

THE SCISSORS

One of the most valuable stretching asanas, the Scissors needs to be held for several minutes to be effective. Among its many benefits is a valuable extension of the sciatic nerve. As ever, the careful, calm mental process is basic.

HOLDING THE POSE

In our fast-paced society, there is a tendency to get things over and done with, but this desire to move on becomes exhausting and creates a feeling of dissatisfaction. One of the pleasures of developing yoga *asanas* is the satisfaction that grows steadily with working slowly and being able to hold static positions for an increasing length of time.

1 Lie on your back, feet together, with the arms stretched out to the sides, palms down. Breathe rhythmically and, as you breathe in, stretch the right leg up into the air.

2 On the out-breath, bring the leg across the body, twisting the hips but keeping the shoulders firmly on the floor. Turn your head to the right as the leg comes down, straight, to the left. Relax as fully as you can and let it come down slowly, aided by the relaxation of a slow out-breath. If the leg does not touch the floor, it does not matter.

Let the rhythm of your breath govern everything: the body will respond and the mind will quiet down. Hold the pose for several minutes, then bring the right leg back, and repeat with the left leg.

THE SCISSORS

11

133

CAT AND DOG

By now you are fully aware of the benefits of the Cat pose. Not only does it benefit the spine and the trunk, it is also a pleasing sensuous movement that makes you feel good. At this stage, you can add the Dog stretch, which benefits legs and ankles.

1 By now, when you do the Cat (see page 24) you are achieving much more spinal movement in the initial process. With the in-breath, drop the back, open the chest and swing up the head and neck.

2 Breathing out, arch the back fully, with the head coming down firmly between the shoulders. Spine and trunk muscles are not only more mobile but the controlled movement strengthens them effectively.

11

Two factors are responsible for a great deal of our back problems: failure to use the trunk effectively and making sudden, jerky movements. The slowly controlled sequence of yoga *asanas* not only enhances mobility of the spine, it also encourages the elasticity of the muscle groups, and promotes overall mobility, including mental agility. The stiffer you are physically, the less likely it is that your brain will work well.

3 After performing the initial movements several times, straighten the legs on an out-breath, thrusting the buttocks into the air.

4 Now bend alternate knees, raising the heel to do so, pressing the other foot firmly against the floor. Leg and ankle muscles are strengthened accordingly.

5 Finally, sink back on to the floor, forehead touching it, the arms lying by the sides, palms up, either side of the feet. Relax for a minute or two.

CAT AND DOG

11

CONTINUING THE PROGRAM

Inverted postures have always played a central role in yoga. That this is natural can be seen from the fact that almost all energetic, healthy children love to do handstands!

There are many reasons for spending a little time upside down; a practical one is providing a useful counter to the constant process of gravity.

Inversion is stimulating, mentally and physically. However, proceed with common sense and, if you have blood pressure or heart problems, consult a well-qualified teacher first.

POSTURES

The Shoulder Stand is sometimes called the Topsy-Turvy pose. By taking your time and establishing a real feeling of mental and physical balance, you can move from a relatively simple position to holding the pose on the shoulders, without the support of the arms. Do remember to keep the shoulders free from tension and let them take the bulk of the weight.

HALF-SHOULDER STAND Page 45

SHOULDER STAND Page 136

POSE OF TRANQUILITY Page 56

The Pose of Tranquility and the Plow also provide a variety of benefits. Maintaining control at all times is most important. Never fall out of these or any other postures. The arms, placed on the ground, provide effective leverage.

PLOW Page 57

CAT   Page 134

DOG   Page 135

The Cat-to-Dog is not strictly an inverted posture, but its value is not dissimilar. Remember how easily and freely cats and dogs stretch. What they can do, you can do too.

The late Swami Sivananda, a doctor before he became a yogi, declared, "It takes 40 muscles to frown and only 15 to smile. Why waste your energy?"

As you become more aware through the practice of yoga, one aspect of this awareness is seeing how energy is wasted. Try to pull a cork out of a bottle and realize how you tense up the muscles of your face, although the latter plays no role in pulling out the cork. This wasted energy seems unimportant at the time, but it adds up. Over any single day you are likely to waste quite a substantial amount, and you wonder why you feel so tired. To achieve the maximum with the least tension, mentally and physically, is central to the art of living.

TRIPOD   Page 132

The Tripod is an important lesson in precision. Forming the equilateral triangle and seeing that the arms make 90° angles are essential. This posture helps greatly in body awareness.

Page 139

MONTH

12

TWELVE

FITTING POSTURE TO NEED

AIMS FOR THE MONTH

It will have become apparent that yoga is not simply a system in which you follow a standard pattern. It is the process of self-realization and, therefore, the principles have to be grasped and then adapted to each individual's needs. As you come to the end of your first year of practice, you should be aware that the development lies in your own approach. While yoga teachers can help, real knowledge lies within you. Through quiet harmony and the development of the capacity to be still, this knowledge becomes apparent.

CONTROLLING STRESS

We have already considered responses to the everyday ups and downs of life; now the time has come to consider this aspect somewhat more deeply. A common statement is, "One person's stress is another person's challenge." We cannot dodge the challenges of life, but we can control our response to them.

While, when life seems to be getting too much for us, we may outwardly seem to be coping, in fact many things are happening at the psychophysical level that can be extremely damaging. Respiration is affected, the body's neuromuscular system is tensed and, in turn, organs are hampered from working properly.

The brain responds according to the most effective impulse it receives. It is for this reason that meditative and visualization techniques have demonstrated human beings' remarkable capacity to achieve calmness even when things seem to be going badly wrong. You can push away the feeling that things are crushing you by sitting and visualizing a beautiful sunrise. You "see" the light appear in the sky, then the sun, slowly making its way into the heavens, with beautiful golden-red light all around. The more you develop this inward picture, the more the feeling of pressure will recede.

Practices such as meditation and visualization apart, *asanas* can be used to overcome mental problems, providing they are approached correctly. If you feel disturbed, for example, remember the Pose of Tranquility (see page 56). Its name describes its purpose and if you push disturbing thoughts away and give yourself to this inverted position, a great feeling of calmness will ensue.

THE THERAPY OF LOVE

The central importance of love in life is
undeniable. Because people tend to
compartmentalize their lives, they often
associate love with human relationships alone
– even just with sexual activity. But there are
no boundaries to love: love of life itself, love
of beautiful things, and love of God are all
aspects of the same central feeling. The effect
of love upon the body is very noticeable: a
person who feels unloved is tense, sharp,
brittle, while someone feeling the emotion of
love is relaxed, soft, and warm. Love is a
much greater experience than that of
immediate relationships, and you can use this
wonderful feeling to enhance your health.
This will, in turn, enhance the feeling!

1 You have already
developed your
performance of the Back
Body Stretch, by
working slowly but
progressively. Now you
move it wholly into the
area of beneficial
visualization. Perform
the posture precisely as
before. When you are as
comfortably stretched as
you can, become aware
of the rhythm of your
breath and, after a
minute or two, see, in
your mind's eye,
someone you love in
front of you and
stretching out his or her
hands to reach yours.
Choose any loving
image: relative, friend,
Jesus Christ, the Lord
Krishna. Stretch forward
to hold the proffered
hands.

The aim in yoga is not to imitate slavishly every technique offered but to absorb the concept and then move into your own realization. Virtually every posture can be linked with visualization to enhance both mental and physical peace and harmony.

2 Let the rhythm of your breath be the flow of your feeling of love. Each time you breathe out, allow your hands to stretch a little further forward. Soon you can feel the sensation of the fingers touching and eventually the grasp of the hands. Lose all consciousness of time. Eventually allow the vision to fade, but allow the sensation of love to remain. Finally, as you breathe in, straighten up, stretching the trunk in the air, before relaxing completely. Mind and body will feel lovingly stretched.

3 As usual, move on into the Cobra. The loving feeling can be enhanced by considering the beauties of nature. For example, bring to mind a fall scene, full of golden tints, and continue looking up at it, allowing your whole body to relax. Again, let the vision fade a little while before you come down on an out-breath and relax.

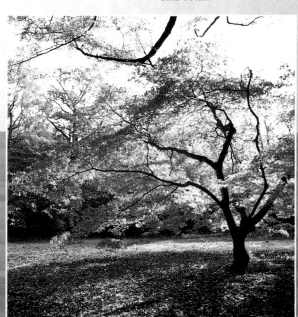

THE THERAPY OF LOVE

12

145

FITTING RELAXATION TO THE NEED

The more you progress in yoga, the more you discover that you have many means of control at your command. Asanas, visualization, meditation are all powerful tools. Relaxation, too, can be developed to enhance general well-being. It is not merely a matter of feeling good, but of actually promoting functions that are truly beneficial.

An immense range of activity is incepted as a result of messages fed to glands in the brain. Central to this activity are the hypothalamus and pituitary glands – sometimes known as the command glands of the body. Interestingly, classical yoga knowledge places a *chakra,* or energy area, at this point. It is given the name *Ajna* and is described as the command *chakra.* As signals, largely based on sensory impulses, are relayed to these glands, so they, in turn, send messages affecting virtually every aspect of our life.

Fight or Flight Response

If the message is alarming, defensive measures are brought into play. When the alarm is intense, the response is described as Fight or Flight, as a preparation for emergency action. The problem is that many unrelieved stress factors trigger aspects of this response without offering a physical form of dissipation, and, as a

Hypothalamus

Pituitary glands

result, changes designed to be helpful become harmful instead. For example, blood sugar, released to promote energy, is not dissipated and can clog the arteries.

Relaxation Response

Other messages to the glands – those of peace and harmony – promote what is termed the Relaxation Response. Calming signals are transmitted through the body which promote balanced, healthy function.

Relaxation is an ideal way of promoting beneficial signals to the command glands. The benefits can be tremendous and far-reaching. Two important areas that have been researched so far are heart disease and high blood pressure, but many equally dangerous problems can be alleviated.

We now know how to lie most effectively in relaxation, keeping the physical tension to a minimum and, as a result, reducing mental tension. In relaxation we play the observer, so, while in this pose, simply bring your awareness to the head and just accept the knowledge that the brain is dealing with a never-ending supply of signals. Be aware, too, that the calmness you are introducing, linked with the peace of the breath, is affecting the response to these signals so that an alarm response becomes a relaxed and peaceful one. This is not as specific as a visualization; it is promoting a general feeling of relaxed well-being, enhanced by the effective relaxed use of the body.

FITTING SOUND TO THE NEED

Many years ago, yogis studied the
importance of sound. You know about the
sound of "Om," called in Sanskrit pranava,
or the primal sound, and the calming effect
this sound creates. Internal sounds can also be
discovered and, while there is obviously a
natural explanation for them, it is amazing
how beneficial they can be. A classical
technique largely cuts out the external senses,
helping us to link more closely with
the internal.

1 Sitting comfortably
erect, place a thumb
firmly against each ear,
blocking out
external sound.

2 Now place the index
fingers over the
closed eyelids, cutting
out sight.

12

Enhancing our awareness is central to an effective life. You need to be conscious of your body, both without and within, in the same way that a managing director, in order to carry out his or her job effectively, needs to have a close knowledge of every aspect of the company's activities. All the different aspects of yoga help you to stay in touch with your body, breath, brain, mind, and consciousness.

3 The second fingers rest against the nostrils, reducing the breath to a very fine and gentle process.

4 The third and fourth fingers cover the top and bottom lips, pressing them together and eliminating speech. Maintain the pressure, keeping a very gentle, fine breath. The result will be an insight into the immense internal activity that you normally never hear, with the throb of the pulse as the "beat." This is a striking reminder of the fact that within us there is an almost continuous factory-like action going on. All these activities are designed to function rhythmically. When we become ill, we talk of disease – in other words, the body has moved out of ease, or its natural rhythm.

If the pressure is continued, eventually a distinguishable sound will be heard, cutting through the "factory" noises. Listening to this brings with it a sense of tranquility.

12

MOVING INTO CONTEMPLATION

Proceeding on the full path of meditation is called Raja Yoga – or the King of the Yogas. The aim is to get ever closer to the union which forms the whole basis of life. While only a few people feel called to explore this path to the fullest, the steps along the way are of tremendous benefit to everyone. For so much of our lives we feel that if we "get by" we are doing well. Yet always there is that nagging feeling at the back of the mind that there is something more – something wonderful to experience. Meditation begins with concentration: the ability to bring the mind to bear exclusively upon one still concept. When this becomes more and more possible (not the same as mastering it wholly), you can move on to contemplation. This can best be described as "becoming a part of."

12

THE ART OF BEING

The concept of living implies action; that of being implies stillness. While we have been born human beings, we might just as well have been a tree, a bird, a flower. In developing the art of contemplation it is sensible to dwell on this thought first. This will make it easier to "be" the rose – or anything else with which you aim to become one.

Many people find that a good object to choose for contemplation is a rose. This is one of the most loved of all flowers. The idea is to visualize a single rose, first taking in the form and the color. Then begin to "see" the shape and linking of every individual petal. At this stage it becomes possible even to appreciate the scent of the rose. The beauty of this flower is such that you can examine it minutely with intense interest. Make sure you have settled on just one bloom – do not move away on to another flower or color.

By continuing the process of this minute examination, you can slowly feel you are becoming a part of the rose. No longer are you an outsider observing; you have merged with it. You have taken on its beauty, you have developed its subtle shape, you are a living rose. This sense of merged identity can continue for some time – there are no limits. When you feel yourself separating once again, become aware of your breath and – very slowly – come back into your own being.

MOVING INTO CONTEMPLATION

12

151

MOVING ON

"The more we learn about the universe, the more it appears to be the product of a single great thought."
**Sir James Jeans,
the eminent British physicist**

Yoga is a process by which we realize more and more fully that we are an integral part of that single great thought.
The end of this book is really just a beginning. A whole new world is in front of you waiting to be explored. Despite the claims of some scientists (by no means all), it is unlikely that we shall learn the entire truth, but there is real joy in unearthing clue after clue and finding they take us closer and closer to this concept of oneness or union which we call yoga. I have enjoyed sharing my experiences with you through this course. Even though our paths may now diverge, the goal remains the same. I wish you joy on your journey.
Howard Kent

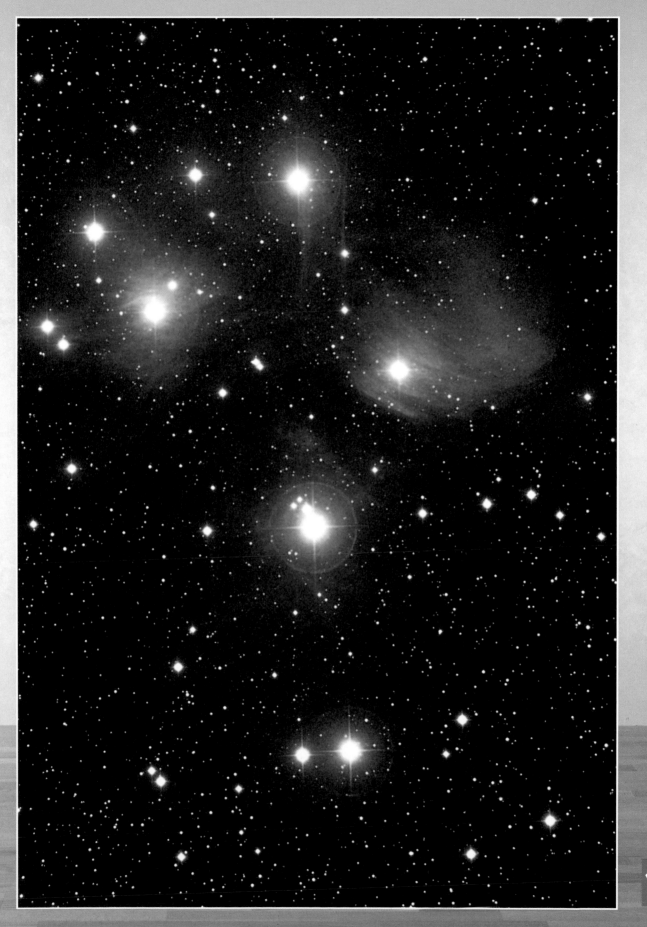

THE LANGUAGE OF YOGA

The early yoga texts were propounded in one of the world's great classical languages, Sanskrit. For a considerable period of time, this was only spoken and the statements were handed down by word of mouth, being memorized and chanted. Subsequently, a written form of Sanskrit appeared, which allowed the texts to be transcribed. There is absolutely no reason why the average student of yoga should seek to master the Sanskrit language, but it is useful to understand the basic terms, especially of the asanas or postures, as some teachers tend to use these exclusively.

The Postures

Posture: *Asana* (ah-sna) This means holding a position.

Bee Breath: *Brahmari*

Lotus Posture: *Padmasana* The best known of the cross-legged positions. This is one of a number of variations.

Sitting on the Heels: *Vajrasana*

Spinal Twist: *Matsyendrasana*

Back Body Stretch: *Paschimotanasana. Paschima* (pashima) means the West. The body is facing the East, so the West side is stretched.

The Cobra: *Bhujangasana*

Relaxation: *Shavasana* The pose of the corpse – that is the totally limp body, after the disappearance of rigor mortis.

Canoe and Reverse Canoe: *Naukasana*

Shoulder Stand: *Sharvangasana*

Fish: *Matsyasana*

Mountain: *Parvatasana*

Plow: *Halasana*

Tree: *Vrikshasana*

Alternate Nostril Breath: *Nadi Shuddan* The cleansing of the subtle nervous system.

Bellows Breath: *Bastrika* **Shining Head Breath:** *Kapalabhati*

Standing Back Body Stretch: *Padhastasana*

Triangle: *Trikonasana*

Bow: *Dhanurasana*

Lion: *Simbhasana*

Hanuman Poses: *Vajrangasana*

(**Note:** In some cases, where there is no agreement on the correct terminology for certain postures, these have been omitted. Similarly, some of the poses shown are not classical yoga and do not have a *Sanskrit* name.)

Other useful terms
Meditation: The sequence of meditation is given as *Dharana* or concentration, *Dhyana* or contemplation and *Samadhi* or the full meditative state, super-consciousness.
Yamas: The way to relate to others – i.e. nonviolently, truthfully, etc.
Niyamas: The way we should relate to ourselves: with equanimity, inner and outer cleanliness, devotion to the creator, etc.

Pratyahara: The ability to control the senses.
Brahmacharya: The ability to overcome lust.
Om: The primal sound of the universe – the all-connecting sound.
Yoga: Oneness, an understanding of the interlinking of everything. Also used to denote a means of reaching such an understanding, as in *Hatha Yoga*.
Chakra: A vortex of energy within the body.
Nadis: The means by which energy flows within the body.

Pronunciation
It should be remembered that in most instances the final "a" is optional: thus, *asana* can also be shown as *asan*. Since *Sanskrit* has both a different alphabet and a different script, for our use it has first to be transliterated into Roman script and then translated. The result is that certain letters vary in pronunciation according to the placing of accents.

CONTINUING YOUR PRACTICE

You will have gathered that yoga is an immense subject and can be tackled in many ways. It is easy to feel somewhat threatened and confused, especially when attempts are made by some teachers to get you to believe their way is the only way.

Yoga is basically very simple: it involves letting unnecessary conditioning drop away. Little children are natural, even innocent, but adults become complex and unnatural. If you use yoga to increase the complexity, you become even more unnatural. Never forget that a technique in yoga is only an aid to reach a goal. The great classical yoga teachers point out that, as you develop on the path, so techniques drop away. The aim, in other words, is not to learn more and more *asanas*, but to understand their purpose and to use them so well that you actually need them less and less.

Never forget that yoga is *self*-realization. Listen to what others – including gurus and teachers – have to say, but remember the final decisions are yours. "To thine own self be true."

Yoga is now practiced virtually throughout the world. There can be relatively few places without a teacher or an organization within reach. There is, however, no single world-wide authority. Generally it will be quite easy to find what is available wherever you live but if you would like help, write to me at this address: Yoga for Health Foundation, Ickwell Bury, Biggleswade, Bedfordshire SG18 9EF, England.

The Foundation operates in many countries and can provide contacts in others. Ickwell Bury is a residential yoga center for those studying yoga and seeking to renew their health. Inquiries always welcome.

OTHER BOOKS FROM THE PEOPLE'S MEDICAL SOCIETY

Take This Book to the Hospital With You
Take This Book to the Gynecologist With You
Take This Book to the Obstetrician With You
Take This Book to the Pediatrician With You
How to Evaluate and Select a Nursing Home
Medicine on Trial
Medicare Made Easy
Your Medical Rights
Getting the Most for Your Medical Dollar
The Consumer's Guide to Medical Lingo
150 Ways to Be a Savvy Medical Consumer
100 Ways to Live to 100
Dial 800 for Health
Your Complete Medical Record
Blood Pressure:
Questions You Have . . Answers You Need
Your Heart:
Questions You Have . . Answers You Need
Arthritis:
Questions You Have . . Answers You Need
Diabetes:
Questions You Have . . Answers You Need
Prostate:
Questions You Have . . Answers You Need
Vitamins and Minerals:
Questions You Have . . Answers You Need
Good Operations – Bad Operations
Test Yourself for Maximum Health
The Complete Book of Relaxation Techniques

INDEX

ACKNOWLEDGMENTS

All images in this book are the copyright of Quarto Publishing plc except for those listed below:

page **36** Life File/Jeremy Hoare; **43** Life File/Miguel Arana; **47** Life File/R Whistler; **49** Life File/Andrew Ward; **53** Life File/ R Whistler; **87** Survival Anglia/J B Davidson; **99**(l) Trip/Eye Ubiquitous; **99**(b) Life File/Fergus Smith; **143** Trip/Helene Rogers; **145** Trip/Roy Styles.

The publishers would like to thank Speedo (Europe) Ltd.